Going Into Labour

'This insightful, thoughtful work needs to be read by all of us who are interested in contemporary childbirth practices. Anna Fielder has brought together the two concepts of labour – work and giving birth – and shows us how both are subsumed under capitalism.'

—Barbara Katz Rothman, author of *In Labor: Women and Power in the Birthplace*

'I have never seen a book that applies Marxist theories and capitalism to childbirth. This book is entirely original and a fascinating read!'

—Robbie Davis-Floyd, cultural, medical and reproductive anthropologist

'Fielder does indeed peel back the layers to reveal how capitalism shapes childbirth. It is refreshing, unique and provides a missing piece in birth scholarship and challenges us to be part of the "collective push to justice and equity".'

—Judith McAra-Couper, Head of School of Clinical Sciences, Auckland University of Technology

'A pivotal addition to Marxist understandings of pregnancy and childbirth. Fielder's nuanced analysis denaturalises human biological reproduction and demonstrates the contradictory features of obstetrics in capitalist society.'

—Kirstin Munro, Assistant Professor of Economics, The New School for Social Research

'Anna Fielder has written the book which midwives and birth activists have long needed as we have struggled with the cumulative damage wrought to birthing environments internationally under the lethal regime of neoliberal capitalism. The resulting acute global shortage of midwives, increasing trauma for women, rising rates of illness and death for the poorest and most marginalised, and the endless nightmare of giving birth in conditions of war and genocide should have every single one of us out on the streets in protest. This book gives us the analytical tools we require to do so effectively.'

—Jo Murphy-Lawless, Centre for Health Evaluation, University of Galway

Mapping Social Reproduction Theory

Series editors Tithi Bhattacharya, Professor of South Asian History and Susan Ferguson, Associate Professor Emerita, Wilfrid Laurier University

Capitalism is a system of exploitation and oppression. This series uses the insights of social reproduction theory to deepen our understanding of the intimacy of that relationship, and the contradictions within it, past and present. The books include empirical investigations of the ways in which social oppressions of race, sexuality, ability, gender and more inhabit, shape and are shaped by the processes of creating labour power for capital. The books engage a critical exploration of social reproduction, enjoining debates about the theoretical and political tools required to challenge capitalism today.

Also available

Social Reproduction Theory:
Remapping Class, Recentering Oppression
Edited by Tithi Bhattacharya

A Feminist Reading of Debt
Luci Cavallero and Verónica Gago

Women and Work:
Feminism, Labour, and Social Reproduction
Susan Ferguson

Disasters and Social Reproduction:
Crisis Response between the State and Community
Peer Illner

Social Reproduction Theory and the Socialist Horizon:
Work, Power and Political Strategy
Aaron Jaffe

Going Into Labour

Childbirth in Capitalism

Anna Fielder

First published 2024 by Pluto Press
New Wing, Somerset House, Strand, London WC2R 1LA
and Pluto Press, Inc.
1930 Village Center Circle, 3-834, Las Vegas, NV 89134

www.plutobooks.com

British Library Cataloguing in Publication Data
A catalogue record for this book is available from the British Library

ISBN 978 0 7453 4949 7 Paperback
ISBN 978 0 7453 4951 0 PDF
ISBN 978 0 7453 4950 3 EPUB

This book is printed on paper suitable for recycling and made from fully managed and sustained forest sources. Logging, pulping and manufacturing processes are expected to conform to the environmental standards of the country of origin.

Typeset by Stanford DTP Services, Northampton, England

Simultaneously printed in the United Kingdom and United States of America

Contents

Acknowledgements

This book has been years in production. Like most human creations, it contains the labour of many. People, conversations and experiences over decades, have influenced the words that it has been possible for me to write over the pages that follow. Particular thanks go to Ciara Cremin and Carisa Showden at the University of Auckland, for their scholarly insights, patience, supervision and friendship over many years.

I am especially grateful to the midwives who, whether in person or from across the seas, have held me, far more than metaphorically, through the different stages of researching and writing. There are more of you than I can possibly name. Special thanks go to Mavis Kirkham, who has always breathed life into mine. Kelly Pidgeon's wisdom, guidance and sense of humour never fail to support me through the many kinds of transition I encounter in life and text-creation. I will leave Mavis and Kelly to decide between them whether I have birthed babies or a book more easily … My colleagues in the AUT Midwifery Department have been patient, wise and supportive as I worked through the final stages of book writing. I am particularly grateful to Teresa Krishnan, whose insights, advice, wisdom and knowledge of Te Ao Māori, have guided me through many paragraphs and sections. Christine Mellor has read, affirmed and verified paragraphs. I thank Jane Evans for her beautiful words, Sara Wickham for long conversations about evidence, and Helen Dresner Barnes for information on insurance. All of you, and more, have shaped the pages of this book.

Barbara Katz Rothman, I cherish the support and advice you have given me over many years, and I look forward to the day that we eventually meet in person. I am particularly grateful to Dr Jade Le Grice at the University of Auckland, for cultural advice through various iterations of this project. Simon Barber, thank you for reading, responding and conversing on specific paragraphs. Kirsten Small, I am indebted for the conversations with you about foetal monitoring – I know you'd spell it differently!

Susan Ferguson's feedback on my writing has been invaluable since before the idea of a book was mooted, and this text has benefitted immeasurably from her insights as series editor. I have also gained hugely from the support and encouragement of series editor Tithi Bhattacharya. Thank you both.

Everyone I have worked with at, and through, Pluto Press, has supported me and been invariably patient: special thanks to David Shulman, Robert Webb and Melanie Patrick. Notwithstanding the input of so many people, any errors that remain are my own.

Sue Bradford, Megan Brady-Clark, Tim Howard, Karen Davis and the Kōtare comrades have provided a political home that I look forward to being more involved with over coming years. Dad, I treasure our conversations about Sheffield working-class history, and your willingness to keep me informed of relevant English news. To Denis, Luqman, Rochana and Simon: thank you for being there.

Warwick's love and ability to 'hold the space' whilst I write, have supported me in more ways than I can say. For that, and all that we share, thank you.

Aaron, Torin and Isla have each, in their own very special ways, reminded me of what is important through the years of research and book writing. With laughs, tears, music, friends, football and much more, they have grown with me on this journey. I could not have asked for better and more inspiring travel-mates.

Mum, this book is for you.

1
Conceiving Childbirth

I must have been about eight years old, sitting cross-legged on the wooden floor of a school assembly. It was the north of England at the end of the 1970s and as was the case each morning the children were gathered together to sing hymns, and to be spoken to about the significance of a particular virtue. That morning's theme, as I remember, was 'labour'. The teacher had asked us to raise our hands if we knew what the word meant. As the daughter of a midwife, I knew about labour. I had been told about the labour that resulted in my arriving in the world by forceps. Years later, I was there when my mother birthed my sister in the back bedroom of our home, and in time I came to understand why she had done that against the advice of doctors. I knew, as the child of any on-call midwife does, that there are no guarantees of when labour will start or end; that it can beckon loved ones in the middle of the day or night; that its outcomes can neither be entirely predicted nor fully controlled; and that, because of that, labour is to be approached with the utmost respect. I knew that labour is a powerful physiological and emotional process; that it can be loud, grunty, painful, raw and euphoric. In that morning assembly, I put my hand up in the air to explain to the school what was meant by the word 'labour', and to this day I am grateful that of all the little hands waving in the air the teacher's gaze did not descend upon mine. The boy who was chosen to explain the meaning of the word labour said that labour is about 'going to work', and the teacher agreed. The assembly moved on, to where I don't recall, but perhaps to ponder on the importance of working hard at school and toiling in the name of the Lord.

Around that time I also came to understand the significance of very different meanings of the word 'labour'. I learned of the labour associated with trade-unionism and with broader political movements for social justice, change and revolution. This is the labour through which people create and produce things, in order to eat, stay warm and survive. I saw that intensely political struggles play out around how the products of that labour are to be shared and distributed – around whether those goods are produced for the meeting of need or the making of profit. In the north of England during my formative years, unemployment was high. Workplaces were closing, leaving streets, families and communities without income. If people could labour at all for a wage, the necessities of their survival were not the primary concern of employers. Just because a life had been spent mining coal did not mean that a miner's home would have enough coal to stay warm through the long strike of 1984–85. Again, I came to understand that labour is to be respected. And you never cross a picket-line.

The social significance of childbirth and the labour of workers were instilled in me from an early age, and these commitments have informed the writing of this book. Through the chapters that follow, an analysis of childbirth is presented which draws upon the work of a figure powerfully associated with the labour of waged workers: Karl Marx. It is an unlikely, if strategic, combining. For all that Marx is known for, his name is not readily associated with the labour of childbirth. Within movements and struggles which take inspiration from the work of Marx, and in which labour is a key focus of political debate, seldom do I hear the labour of childbirth discussed, if mentioned at all. Having worked as a midwife and given birth three times, I am also involved in spaces where the politics of childbirth (the funding of perinatal services, the treatment of people within such spaces, the working conditions of health and birth workers, etc.) is a mainstay of action, activism and conversation. In environments where childbirth is the primary focus of concern, references to Marx are most notable by their absence. With respect to these two seemingly diverse strands of my life – Marxism and the politics of birth – it has long concerned me that never the twain shall meet. I began the research upon which much of this book is based over six years ago, inspired by a commitment to ensuring that the twain of Marxism and of childbirth *do* meet, and that conversations about the significance and potentials of such entwining can develop. Much has changed since then.

To some extent this is a timely text. Historically, birth workers are not eminently associated with industrial action, yet over recent years they have been on strike in a range of countries. When members of the midwifery trade union in the UK voted to strike in 2014, it was the first time that they had done so during the lifetime of the organisation, which dates back to 1881.[1] In Aotearoa New Zealand, where I have written this manuscript, midwives and nurses have protested in the streets many times over the past few years.[2] Pay and working conditions are primary concerns. Birth workers were already leaving their jobs in droves before coronavirus became a household word. Employment conditions worsened during the COVID-19 pandemic, and the haemorrhaging of skilled workers has continued. Those who exit their jobs speak of financial pressures but more significant for some is the frustration, anxiety and sheer sadness of being unable to do the work they love to do. Some are finding it impossible in current conditions to provide birth care that is *safe* and *supportive*: that is to say, to provide birth *care* at all.[3]

The United States has been described as the most dangerous country in the so-called 'developed world' in which to give birth, whilst also being one of the most expensive.[4] Even prior to the COVID-19 pandemic the US maternal mortality rate had been rising, and was well above that of other comparatively high-income countries.[5] In 2021, the US maternal mortality rate continued to rise, with Black women far more likely to die of pregnancy and birth-related causes than white women.[6] Maternal death is described as the 'tip of the iceberg' in so far as the dangers haunting childbirth are concerned, not only in the US.[7] Many people – infants and adults – have pregnancy-related pathologies, or have been harmed, injured and/or traumatised through experiences in the perinatal services. Some of those injuries endure across lifetimes.

There have undoubtedly been improvements in birthing conditions over recent decades – at least for some people. Routine episiotomies (cuts to a person's perineum *as a matter of course* when they are giving birth) are no longer practiced in many hospitals. Gone are the days when all babies were hung upside-down at birth and slapped on the back by eager doctors. There is increased institutional support for the closest support networks of pregnant people – their families, partners and/or friends – to stay with them as they labour and birth (at least that was the case prior to the COVID-19 pandemic). Many people state that they are satisfied with the pregnancy and birth care that they receive, although significant proportions are not. There have been wider positive developments, some of which are discussed in later chapters, but there continues to be vast scope for improving pregnancy and birth care. In addition to the need for improvements in maternal death rates, particularly for Women of Colour, there is a significant need for improvements in preterm (premature) birth rates. In 2023, the World Health Organization described the world as 'flat-lining' on preventing preterm birth rates over the past decade, and in some parts of the world rates have been rising.[8] There is a global shortage of midwives, and even if that were addressed there is considerable scope for improving the ways in which birth care is structured – some might say delivered – in many institutions. As events around childbirth can have lifetime implications for entire families and across generations, the effects of improvements in birth services are far-reaching. Whilst there have been some encouraging policy developments, positive change within pregnancy and birth care often feels slow-paced at best. 'What is holding back global progress?' enquire both workers and academics from across the world.[9] A key premise of this book is that analyses of childbearing must grapple with the role of capitalism, if they are to account for why calls for change in relation to childbirth often go apparently unheeded.

It would be unfair and inaccurate to suggest that there are *no* references to capitalism within the birthing literature.[10] There are, and I sense that the word appears more frequently in recent publications than was the case a few years ago. Yet it remains the case that discussion of capitalism is not prevalent within the literature that many birth workers read on a regular basis. This is so to the extent that in 2024 an article appeared in the UK *Midwifery Matters* journal in which a midwife reflected on whether there is 'some sort of ban on the word "capitalism" in writing around birth'.[11] If there is, responsibility for such relative silence cannot be placed entirely with those who work or are activists in the field of childbirth. The tradition which produced the most powerful and enduring critiques of capitalism – that is to say, Marxism – has not habitually been forthcoming in developing analyses of birth. Nor am I alone in noting a paucity of Marxist work on the topic of human childbearing. At the end of the 1970s, Raymond Williams spoke of the failure of Marxists to develop comprehensive analyses of this aspect of human life process:

> It is very remarkable that if you look across the whole gamut of Marxism, the material-physical importance of the human reproductive process has been generally overlooked. Correct and necessary points have been made about the exploitation of women or the role of the family, but no major account of this whole area is available. Yet it is scarcely possible to doubt the absolute centrality of human reproduction and nurture and the unquestioned physicality of it.[12]

When I first began researching parturition through Marxism, it seemed to me that little had changed since Williams spoke those words decades ago. Even in much of the literature which sits within the broad rubric of Marxist-feminism, references to childbirth appeared relatively infrequent. Biological reproduction was gestured towards from time to time, primarily in passing. When discussions of reproductive rights feature within the canons of Marxist feminism, the focus tends to be upon abortion and contraception. Access to knowledge, techniques and services which enable people to safely prevent and/or end pregnancies are a vital component of any equitable society now or in the future. Yet that is only part of the story as far as so-called 'biological reproduction' is concerned.

THE CONTRADICTORY TERRAIN OF CHILDBIRTH

Globally, around 300,000 maternal deaths are linked to pregnancy and birth each year.[13] The vast majority of these are preventable. In order to reduce maternal deaths across the world, the access that many people have to emergency procedures such as caesarean section must be considerably improved. This is not least the case in sub-Saharan Africa, where many people experience a serious 'lack of access to this lifesaving surgery'.[14] In order to protect the lives and health of childbearing people and babies, there is also a need to prevent uncomplicated labours across the world from becoming complicated as a result of unnecessary medical procedures which cause more harm than good and, integral to that, suboptimal care. Whilst caesarean sections can be a life-saving procedure, they are also associated with higher rates of many adverse sequelae than are vaginal births. The possibility of somebody experiencing an adverse reaction to the anaesthetic or inadvertent surgical damage to their bladder, cannot be ruled out. A primary caesarean introduces a scar into a person's uterus which can create complications in future pregnancies, including increasing the likelihood of ectopic pregnancy, rupture of the uterus and complications at the site of the placenta.[15] Globally, elective caesareans – that is to say, caesareans which take place before a person goes into labour – are associated with phenomena as diverse as raised rates of maternal infection, of respiratory complications for the baby and of neonatal mortality.[16] If such infections and respiratory complications cannot be easily treated or responded to, consequences can be fatal. Given such concerns, researchers and commentators currently emphasise the need within pregnancy and birth care, to move beyond scenarios in which some people receive 'too little too late' and others 'too much too soon'.[17] Both are problematic.

I emphasise this at an early stage of the book because it has been widely presupposed that as medical interventions developed, birth became safer. In some ways this has been so, yet not necessarily for the reasons assumed. In advanced capitalist countries, mortality rates associated with pregnancy fell considerably over the five decades which ended in the 1980s.[18] In England and Wales, they were comparatively constant from the first collection of national statistics in 1838 until the mid-1930s when they began to rapidly improve.[19] Rather than 4.2 maternal deaths per 1,000 births at the beginning of the twentieth century, by the late 1970s/early 1980s, there were 0.12 deaths per 1,000 births.[20] Lines of causality are far from linear and are notoriously difficult to prove. The introduction of pharmaceuticals to treat bacterial infections (specifically sulphonamides) in the mid-1930s appears to have had a pivotal impact on the maternal death rate in England.[21] Innovations such as the development of penicillin, ergometrine (to control post-birth haemorrhage) and improved access to blood transfusions are also seen as contributing factors.[22] Yet to unequivocally equate reduced death rates with medical intervention is a categorical mistake. Maternal mortality rates have historically been high in localities where 'maximum surgical interference' was common as a so-called 'prophylactic' (preventative) measure.[23] In the nineteenth and twentieth centuries, doctors often used forceps in what were otherwise straightforward labours, thereby introducing into childbearing bodies surgical lacerations that were highly vulnerable to fatal infection. Before the new anti-bacterial treatments were introduced in the 1930s, infection (puerperal sepsis) was indeed a primary killer of new mothers and had been for some time.[24] That was the case to some extent *because* of high levels of forceps deliveries and inadequate antiseptic practices. There is a powerful argument that before the mid-1930s, maternity care was having a *detrimental* effect in many localities and the introduction of the anti-bacterial sulphonamides was able to mask or cover that up, at least to some extent.[25] To attribute sole responsibility for lowered maternal death rates with medical intervention, is to render invisible the twists, turns, contradictions and tragedies which haunt the history and ongoing practices of childbirth.

SHIFTING CONTOURS OF ANALYSIS

Over recent decades, academics and activists have attributed responsibility for many of the problems which developed in relation to childbirth, to a range of social forces. The rise in caesarean sections and use of heavily routinised care with iatrogenic effects have been seen as a product of industrialism or industrial society.[26] Patriarchal power structures have also been held to account.[27] It is now widely documented that prior to the eighteenth century, women in Europe as well as North America had given birth largely in their homes supported by other women, friends, relatives and midwives. By various mechanisms, which differed between countries and localities, the influence of male doctors grew. Women were largely excluded from becoming physicians and were prohibited by tradition or other means from wielding instruments such as forceps which doctors increasingly deployed.[28] By the mid-to-late twentieth century, and earlier in many places, childbirth had been constituted as a medical event and was taking place primarily in hospitals: in other words, on the terrain of 'medical men'. Childbearing has been described as undergoing a process of appropriation by men even well beyond the mid-twentieth century. Yet over recent years, there has been growing acknowledgement that much feminist research carried out on people's experiences of childbearing has centred the experiences of white, often middle-class, cis women. In highlighting the patriarchal character of birth-care institutions – of their staffing structures and prevalent clinical practices – social and historical forces and determinants of health such as racism and colonisation, have often been overlooked.

In Aotearoa New Zealand, Māori are tangata whenua, the people of the land. The relationship of the Indigenous people of Aotearoa with the land is crucial to Māori knowledge of birth and creation. In Te Ao Māori (the Māori world) it is from the land – Papatūānuku, the earth mother – that all things and people are born.[29] The word whenua denotes both land and placenta in the Māori language, and through the Indigenous practice of whenua ki te whenua (burying and returning the whenua to the land) 'the relationship between the newborn child and the land of their birth' is supported and reinforced.[30] Land is also nourished.[31] Through processes of colonisation, the colonisers claimed land as their own; Indigenous kinship and family structures were disrupted,[32] and traditional childbearing practices eroded.[33] By the middle decades of the twentieth century, when many Māori women were entering hospitals to give birth, even the deeply significant practice of whenua ki te whenua was prevented, as hospital policies and practices instructed the disposal and incineration of whenua (placentas) through institutional mechanisms.[34] As Māori are today remaking traditional birthing practices, pregnancy and birthing are important and powerful sites of decolonisation.

Although the precise contours of birthing landscapes vary from one location to another, structural racism is deeply engrained across national – as well as international – contexts. In the UK, data from 2019–21 demonstrates that Black women are almost four times more likely than white women to die during pregnancy and the six weeks that follow birth.[35] For women of Asian ethnic backgrounds, the likelihood is two times that of white birthing people. Across the Atlantic in the US, the maternal mortality ratio between 2007 and 2016 was highest for Black women, followed by American Indian and Alaska Native women (combined figure).[36] In some states, rates of maternal death are particularly high for specific racialised groups. In 2019 in New York City, Black women were nine times more likely to die of pregnancy-related causes than were white women.[37] Today, work to reduce maternal mortality rates and to increase the numbers of midwives and doulas of colour (doulas being specialists providing non-clinical support to people through and after pregnancy, and sometimes around death), are struggles also against racism, white supremacy and the ongoing effects of colonisation.

The birthing literature contains scattered references to *specific features* of capitalism: to commodification, commercialisation, economic barriers, or economic drivers, for example. To give an example, the editors of a special edition of the *Health, Risk & Society* journal comment that the issue 'highlights the analytical relevance of the influence of economic drivers within the governance of reproductive processes, in that financial or market concerns seem to increasingly shape risk discourses and practices'.[38] Various academics have pondered the effects of neoliberalism upon birth. Towards the end of the 1990s in Australia, neoliberal administrative measures to boost private health insurance coverage are reported to have increased wealthy women's access to private obstetricians.[39] Yet analysis considering reified aspects of political-economy such as *economic barriers* to healthcare, or investigation at the level of neoliberalism, does not in and of itself demand reference to or critique of capitalism. In other words, aspects of capitalism might be honed in upon without mention of the system to which they are integral. In her political-economy of birth in the US, Barbara Bridgman Perkins observed that twentieth-century approaches to medical service provision could indeed be described as '*capitalist*' but she was concerned that the word carries considerable 'baggage' and spoke of finding the word '*business*' more useful and 'generally applicable'.[40] Perkins' work is important in emphasising the significance of political-economy in an arena where the influence of political-economy has seldom been acknowledged by activists and those seeking progressive change. Yet if the c-word that is capitalism cannot be uttered in relation to birth care, there is a danger that capitalism itself becomes further naturalised, like water to the proverbial fish.

When the words 'capitalist' or 'capitalism' do appear within the birthing literature, they perhaps feature most prevalently in relation to the US medical system where private enterprise and competition are profoundly entrenched in healthcare provision. For instance, midwife Jennie Joseph says of US maternity care: 'It is a capitalist system, it is a business model.'[41] She adds, 'we are making a business of obstetrics rather than a practice of obstetrics.'[42] I agree, and birth care is also entrenched within capitalism well beyond the US. Outside of the United States, social scientists and birth writers have indicated that capitalism operates as a background context for developments within birthing environments.[43] Australian midwife Sally Tracy contends that over recent years 'we have lived through tumultuous waves of change in global economic thinking and behaviour so that any evaluation of maternity services in terms of sustainability and cost should be viewed within the current broader economic and political context.'[44] She gestures towards that wider environment as 'The end of the "golden years" – the crisis of capitalism'.[45] My contention is that there is need for far more analysis of childbirth within the context of capitalism – be that capitalism in the present or the past. I therefore hope that this book will contribute towards a conversation that is already happening but that could be further amplified and developed.[46] In this respect, I am particularly inspired by the publication of a 2024 special edition of the *History of the Present* journal, in which childbearing is unambiguously placed in the context of racial capitalism.

INTRODUCING CAPITALISM (THIS IS ONLY PART OF THE STORY)

Through the pages of this text, I develop an analysis of childbirth in capitalism, and I draw upon Marx's understanding of capitalism in order to do so. Marx saw capitalism as involving far more than trade or the exchange of goods in the market place. As Ellen Meiksins Wood emphasises, almost since time began people have made money through 'buying cheap and selling dear'.[47] That is not what capitalism is about. She describes capitalism as:

> … a system in which goods and services, down to the most basic necessities of life, are produced for profitable exchange, where even human labour-power is a commodity for sale in the market, and where all economic actors are dependent on the market.[48]

It is important to emphasise that, for Marx, such a system could not have been normalised and consolidated until land was taken from the people who worked that land (see Chapter 2). That process of appropriation happened in different ways in different places, but once people no longer had access to land on which they could grow crops for their survival, most had no option but to sell their capacity to work – their 'labour power' – in return for money (a wage). The masses increasingly worked to produce the goods needed to survive by earning a wage from employers (broadly speaking the capitalist class who privately owned land and used it for purposes such as commercial agriculture, sites of manufacturing, etc.), and then purchasing the necessities of survival with their wage. If this were simply a case of production and exchange being mediated by money, it *might* not be problematic. However capitalists must also eat and live to survive, and they must make profit so that they can invest in their own enterprises and remain competitive in the future. As the above quotation from Meiksins Wood indicates, within capitalism even the most basic goods are produced in order to facilitate 'profitable exchange'. Marx was interested in how that profit is made – and he contended that the processes and relations which facilitate such profit-making involve adversity for many.

He ascertained that in capitalism workers on aggregate must produce goods of more value (broadly speaking worth) than the value (worth) of their wages. When that happens, capitalists can sell products for more than they paid for them to be produced. The extra (surplus-value) appears in the form of money when goods produced are sold by capitalists in the marketplace. Some of the money will be spent by capitalists on such items as goods (including luxury goods) for their own consumption, but they will invest a considerable amount of it into their businesses as capital.[49] This is important because if they are to survive as capitalists, they need to purchase such things as new machinery and technology (perhaps to increase productivity or facilitate product-line expansion), bigger premises (allowing economies of scale), etc. Marx also saw that it is not in the interests of capital to raise wages above the level that is socially necessary, or to employ more workers than are absolutely required, as to do so would curtail the quantity of surplus-value produced. For him, capitalism therefore requires the relentless pursuit of surplus-value in conditions where many people simply do not have the means to purchase the goods produced. Partly for this reason, he stressed, the system is frenetically driven and inherently unstable. Capitalism is like a 'sorcerer' who is unable to 'control the powers of the nether world whom he has called up by his spells'.[50]

This is of course an oversimplification of Marx's understanding of capitalism and some aspects of his work have been challenged, even by those who could easily be categorised as Marxist. Other features of Marx's analysis have been expanded upon, and much has changed since he was writing in the nineteenth century. Nonetheless, his work provides insights which remain incredibly pertinent to this day. The world is certainly no less crisis-ridden than it was 150 years ago, and is probably more so. There has been rapid expansion of goods, technology, infrastructure and commodities, and these have permeated almost all areas of life. That is *not to say* that everybody has equal access to these. The gap between rich and poor is growing wider, and none of this would be alien to Marx. Although he was of the view that capitalism's days were far more numbered than they turned out to be, many of the developments that people are grappling with today can be made sense of by drawing, and perhaps expanding, upon Marx's nineteenth-century analysis of capitalism. In so far as childbirth is concerned, there has been rapid proliferation of birthing technologies over recent decades, but still many people cannot access even the basics of safe birth (such as a safe caesarean section if required). Even health services and birthing facilities that people do not pay for at the point of use – those that are funded, for instance, through general taxation – are stocked with technologies and pharmaceuticals that were produced and sold for profit. In the words of a political economist who sits firmly within the Marxist tradition, health services of that kind are far from immune to being 'plundered by private pharmaceutical monopolies or semi-monopolies'.[51] In the UK, which has a publicly owned health system, the creeping privatisation of healthcare has been afoot for some time. Health workers are under pressure, and it would be naïve to assume that this does not affect the support and care of childbearing people. Across many countries, industrial action by birth workers is demonstrative of inadequate pay and inadequate staffing. Birth workers tend not to take strike action unless they absolutely must, indicating the extent of their discontent and concern. Given the range of crises which beleaguer pregnancy and birthing services, there is plenty of theoretical rationale for drawing creatively upon the work of Marx in order to analyse the dynamics of contemporary childbirth. In fact, it surprises me that Marx's work is not referred to more often in order to do so.

There is also an element of historical fortuity in the writing of this book. During the years of twentieth-century neoliberalism, the name of Marx was arguably more profaned than the word 'capitalism'. In few circles could Marx be mentioned without conversation being swallowed by anxieties of Stalinist-type dictatorship. It is feasible, and in my view *necessary*, to denounce authoritarian rule *without* wholesale rejection of Marx's analysis of capital. Conversations on this seldom appeared possible towards the end of the twentieth century, symptomatic perhaps of the prevailing neoliberal climate. Twenty or so years later, vast edifices of wealth, illusion and attempts at sheer survival, came tumbling down in the 2008 financial crisis. In even the most privileged and celebrated enclaves of capitalist success, many lost bricks, mortar, jobs and futures. Capitalism was shown to be far from the stable panacea that many had assumed it to be. Generations of people who had never learned about Marx, began scrambling to make sense of the devastating and unpredictable environment in which they found themselves.[52] The work of Marx was reached for anew. Marx, it has been said, is back. If we are to grapple with the vast array of challenges facing the world today, we must – I argue – create an environment in which he is encouraged to stay.

NOTES ON METHOD

There are different ways in which I could have approached the writing and structuring of this book. If one assumes that Marx developed an overarching theoretical schema for application in any situation, childbirth might have been squeezed into such an analytic framework: pregnant people could have been cast as impoverished workers struggling for control of the means of re-production whilst their labour processes are presided over in minute detail by capitalist-cum-obstetric figures who derive profit in the process. That may not be an entirely inaccurate analogy, particularly in countries where birthing services are provided primarily by commercial businesses. Yet as discussed in the next chapter, situating childbearing people purely as workers for capital veils much of the nuance, contradiction and diversity of contemporary childbearing labours and subjectivities. Marx did not develop a meta-theoretical framework for universal application, into which childbirth might be singularly slotted. My own approach to the analysis of childbirth in capitalism, as presented in Chapters 3–6 of this book, takes inspiration from Marx's notes on method. In order to explain this attention to method, a brief and preliminary detour into the notion of nature in birth is helpful …

In the 1980s, American Marxist Fredric Jameson observed that capital had undergone such a remarkable expansion into previously uncommodified areas, that a 'radical eclipse of Nature itself' had taken place.[53] Today I am certainly not keen on saying that childbirth is 'natural'. As a prominent US sociologist of birth has observed, 'one would be hard put to claim that anything people do is "natural"'.[54] The term 'natural birth' is notoriously 'slippery' and used to denote an array of birthing experiences, ranging from labours which do not involve a caesarean section to entirely unmedicated births, with much in between and beyond.[55] Yet however 'slippery' the natural may be, through the twentieth century and into the twenty-first, there has been much yearning for the natural in birth – and perhaps understandably so. Calls for natural birth have served as powerful and reverberating rallying cries mobilising people in resistance to intense, often indiscriminate, medicalisation. Whether notions of natural childbirth are helpful or not, undiscerning medical practice (often facilitated by medical-tech produced and manufactured for profit rather than health) is decidedly *not.* Many of the diverse groups and movements often implied by the umbrella term 'natural birth movement' have – through decades of the twentieth century and beyond – challenged the effects of social forces that must, in my view, be called into question. Yet such movements have also been shaped and influenced by some of the very same social forces and relations that produced the intense medicalisation they were opposing. For instance, Grantly Dick-Reed was an obstetrician and early advocate of 'natural childbirth' who wrote a book with that title; he described the childbearing mother as a *factory*, adding that 'by education and care she can be made more efficient' both in parturition and in 'the art of motherhood'.[56] He saw his techniques for natural childbirth as a means of maximising the efficiency of that factory. It is intriguing (one might say revealing) imagery from a figure who was inspirational in a movement that is often seen as having lauded nature and that even pitted itself against processes of industrialisation.

Over the duration of a few twentieth-century decades, many books, including Dick-Reed's own, were published and education programmes developed advocating a range of strategies and techniques for achieving, or associated with, 'natural birth'. It is a contradiction now deeply embedded in the landscape of childbearing, that the word 'natural' was used to depict approaches to birthing that involved considerable education, training and *work*: practices that are, in short, profoundly social.[57] Sociologist Ann Oakley was acutely aware of this, and of problems associated with what she called 'the idealization of "natural" childbirth'.[58] If the natural had been turned into a thing, an end product – an ideal – to be worked towards and achieved (one that, if unattained, might contribute to some women feeling inadequate and ashamed[59]), there were also wider dynamics operating. Hospitals in the US, aware that their own medicalised offerings were not entirely palatable to key sectors of the population, began to advertise and promote their services through images of 'natural birth'.[60] In time, the 'idealized birth experience' is said to have been transformed 'into a commodity for both patient-consumers and attendant-providers'.[61] So-called 'natural birth' is today associated with a range of commodified paraphernalia, from aromatherapy oils, birthing balls and soft lighting, to birth pools and commercial childbirth classes. Writer on human biotechnology Marcy Darnovsky contends that the primary twenty-first-century 'purveyors of the naturalistic fallacy' are 'marketers of breakfast cereals, cosmetics, and prenatal vitamins'.[62] Renditions of the 'natural' are crucial marketing strategies in promoting commodities produced in surplus-value producing factories across the world. Through such mechanisms, natural birth has been configured as something to not only aim towards, work for, achieve, or desire, but also to orientate one's consumer spending towards and perhaps even (attempt to) purchase. This is important as, although the term 'natural birth' is still used in some birthing circles, today many birth practitioners and activists who might be dubbed and/or criticised (not least on media platforms) as proponents of natural birth do not use that terminology at all. Many speak instead of providing support for physiological birthing processes or use a range of other (still shifting) terminology. In short, yearnings for – and renditions of – 'the natural' in birth can be read, at least in part, as bound up, in and with, a wide range of forces and dynamics integral to capitalism, which played out through the twentieth century and continue to do so.

If 'nature' in birth has been reified – assumed to constitute a coherent object or entity – and invested with economic deliberations and financial imperatives, it is far from alone in that respect. A key premise of this book is that the making of profit and the accumulation of capital have driven the consolidation and actualisation of many of the most prominent features of contemporary birthing environments. Ideas, concepts and features of the birthing landscape that are highly normalised have often been consolidated and reified in ways which support the accumulation of capital. Through the central chapters of this book, I draw upon Marx's methodological approach in order to illustrate how this has been, and continues to be, so.

In his few comments on method in political economy, Marx wrote of the ways in which aspects of life which appear most immutable or 'natural' often do so as an effect of the consolidation of intensely social forces, relations and elements. He was musing over how seventeenth-century scholars had come to understand their field of study. They commenced their investigations at the level of the nation, the population, the state, or a collection of states. These were obvious starting points for research, as they were highly normalised social formations: Marx described them as 'the real and the concrete'.[63] He saw that scholars beginning with these features as points of analytic departure invariably identified a range of relations and abstractions that combined within the initial starting point(s); these included division(s) of labour, money, etc.[64] In this respect, the points of analytic departure appeared as obvious places to start investigation precisely *because* they were aggregates of many other 'determinations and relations'.[65] This reminds me of metaphorical ants to an ant-hill: the 'thing' that is most visible and obvious exists as an effect of a range of constitutive elements and relations. Moreover, Marx saw that different concrete starting points are related to one another within the much broader environment of which they are a part. Once those – as well as the multiple 'conceptions and relations' which combine within them – are all taken into account, analysis can open out to the level of a much broader system: one of 'international exchange' and the 'world market'.[66] Global capitalism is, in short, a complex and dynamic ensemble – a 'totality' to use his terminology – of many different aspects which interrelate. Perhaps it is not surprising therefore, that political-economist David Harvey has used the term 'ecosystemic' to describe capitalism.[67] Some features of the ecosystem are more visible and prominent than others, yet even the most salient aspects do not exist or operate in isolation from others.

Marx's work is seen to mark an analytic departure from prevalent – particularly 'empiricist or neo-positivist' – understandings of abstraction and of associated interpretations of what terms such as 'material' or 'concrete' mean.[68] His use of the word 'concrete' does not indicate an arena of (impenetrable) physical matter nor of purely sense experience. Neither does he understand abstraction as relating to disembodied ideas or concepts. Whilst people's existence, experiences and needs can be intensely corporeal, it is through ideas and language that humans make sense of the world, and for Marx, ideas operate with most *gravitas* and force – they come to *matter* so to speak – when they are the effect of many well-established social relations, forces and elements. In drawing upon Marx's method for inspiration, I have not given particular focus in this book to the physicality – the flesh and blood, so to speak – of birthing bodies. Instead, I emphasise key categories and concepts which carry weight and heft, which command attention, within contemporary mainstream birthing environments (by which I mean, primarily, the so-called 'maternity' services). These are categories that are so normalised in such contexts that they tend to appear neutral and pass unnoticed. I have sought to unravel these prevailing categories – to 'peel back the layers' so to speak – in order to identify the relations and dynamics integral to capitalism which support them to assume the authority and form that they currently do. In this way, the operations of global capitalism which currently influence and shape childbirth, can be drawn to the foreground for consideration.

As a result of my reading and, doubtless, personal experience, I settled on obstetric *technology*, *risk*, *evidence* and *choice* (that is, choice on the part of birthing people) as concrete starting points for the analysis developed in the central chapters of this book. Testimony to the 'concrete' nature of these phenomena, it often felt as if they chose themselves as starting points for analysis. For instance, contemporary birthing units are filled with a vast array of equipment and technologies: electronic foetal monitors, ultrasound scanners, surgical instruments, syringes, drips, drip-stands, a growing range of pharmaceuticals, electronically adjustable beds, surgical tables, and far more. Medical and related journals contain information on the latest technologies and approaches for using them. Interestingly, Darnovsky has observed that criticisms of the 'natural' in pregnancy all too often presuppose a correlative 'deference to the technological'.[69] In so far as this is the case, perhaps there is a lurking, painful grain of truth underpinning the Monty Python skit about 'the machine that goes PING!' – deference to the machine predominates, over and above consideration of the childbearing person, even if the machine has little if any function in relation to childbirth.[70] This book would have certainly felt incomplete without consideration of the significance of technology within contemporary childbirth.

Risk is also omnipresent within contemporary birthing spaces. Even the healthiest of pregnancies tend to be defined in terms of risk, and a glance through most medical, midwifery, nursing, or birth activist publications will reveal countless references to *risk*: to the identification, assessment, mediation and management thereof. 'Is it even possible to talk about pregnancy and childbirth in language other than that of risk?' enquires sociologist of birth Barbara Katz Rothman.[71] *Evidence* as a concrete feature of the birthing landscape rose to prominence in the 1990s, and today many would consider it irresponsible for people to make decisions about childbirth that are *not* supported by evidence. In this context, evidence is information obtained through scientific clinical and/or epidemiological research, and towards the end of the twentieth century, the Randomised Controlled Trial (RCT) was heralded as the 'gold standard' – the most robust form – of evidence to inform decision-making in healthcare settings. Testimony to the concrete character of RCTs, they were deemed the standard by which all other forms of evidence were to be judged. Then there is *choice*. Be it consumer choice, patient choice, informed choice, women's choice, or other varieties of choice, renditions of choice (and the absence thereof) have become pivotal in defining the quality and character of contemporary birthing care. In this book, a chapter each is dedicated to exploring *technology*, *risk*, *evidence* and *choice* respectively.

Through researching and writing for this manuscript, I have come to refer to the rather unruly ensemble of technology, risk, evidence and choice as 'TREC'. Many pregnant people, particularly in advanced capitalist countries, find themselves navigating and exploring – trekking through and across – these apparently neutral features of the birthing landscape, as they embark on their pregnancy journeys. Whilst other features of contemporary birthing could be emphasised, my ongoing conversations with birth workers indicate that technology, risk, evidence and choice are solid places to start. Separately and together, the constituent elements of TREC have come to play a crucial role in defining, as well as structuring and regulating, the activities and movements of many childbearing people and of paid birth workers. This is not least the case in advanced capitalist contexts where English is an official language, such as the US, Aotearoa New Zealand and the UK. The central chapters of this book are focused primarily upon birth in these lands, although I also draw upon important examples and literature from Ireland, Canada, Australia and a range of other countries. Some aspects of the analysis may also be relevant beyond those contexts.

This book's primary (albeit not exclusive) emphasis upon birth in English-speaking countries – particularly evident in Chapters 3 to 6 – emerged largely due to practical considerations pertaining to my own experience(s) and to the availability of relevant literature in the language I read most fluently. The history of British imperialism (one of the conduits through which the influence of capital spread across the world) in relation to those countries lurks in the background of that context. That said, the maternity care systems in different countries have important differences and specificities, and in covering key features of childbirth across a range of countries, the analysis developed through the chapters of this book is wide-reaching. In so being, my hope is that it provides plenty of scope for future research projects and empirical studies to drill down into some of the details (perhaps of local regulations or specific service structures) that are, by necessity, unmentioned or unexplored in this book. Once capitalism is firmly and unambiguously acknowledged, and widely recognised, as shaping contemporary perinatal care in manifold ways, any number of studies potentially become possible to explore and interrogate the empirical details of such dynamics. Rather than regional and localised birthing arrangements – and activism even – being analysed as primarily discrete or isolated phenomena, they might be analysed for the possibility that they comprise 'many determinations and relations', some of which are integral to the heaving totality that is global capitalism.

OVERVIEW OF THE CHAPTERS

If this book was inspired by an assumption that Marxists have been silent on the topics of pregnancy and childbirth, that presupposition was not entirely accurate. In Chapter 2, I introduce and expand upon various aspects of Marx's theory, whilst also considering some of the ways in which gestation and birth have been presupposed, and at times directly discussed, within the historical materialist tradition. The text can be read as a 'bringing together' of various conversations within Marxism, with a particular focus upon how childbearing features in those discussions. Thereby demonstrated are some of the ways in which Marx and others who followed in his footsteps have 'denaturalised' a range of presuppositions and categories that are integral to capitalism, and have referred to pregnancy and/or childbearing as they did. For instance, over recent years Marxist-feminists have directly reflected upon the emergence of the global surrogacy industry in which people are paid to gestate and birth babies with whom they have no genetic link. In conditions such as these, powerful assumptions regarding what it means to be a *mother* and the *nature* of families are being contested. Such challenges to prevailing conceptions and configurations of familial formations are inseparable from the very processes of capitalist expansion. In the words of Sophie Lewis, 'Pregnancy work is not so much disappearing or getting easier as crashing through various regulatory barriers onto an open market. Let the poor do the dirty work, wherever they are cheapest (or most convenient) to enrol.'[72] Yet well beyond pregnancy as financially reimbursed employment, childbirth is heavily imbued with the logics and relations of capital. That, rather than gestational surrogacy, is the focus of this book.

This book has been written with at least two sets of readers in mind: those with an interest in Marxism and those with a specific interest in childbirth. These are not entirely distinct or discrete groups, but if Chapter 2 is more accessible to those who are well versed in Marxist theory, others may prefer to focus their reading from Chapter 3. That is the first chapter in which I hone in on a specific element of the TREC ensemble: obstetric technologies. In a 2012 survey of 2,400 people who gave birth in the US, 87 per cent of respondents experienced birthing with one or more of the following technologies: instrumental delivery (forceps or ventouse [suction]), pharmacological augmentation (speeding-up) of labour, a caesarean section, epidural analgesia, or an attempted (medical) induction of labour.[73] In the UK context, Ann Oakley indicates that between research she carried out in the mid-1970s and a similar study some 30 years later, the use of pregnancy ultrasound scans, caesarean section and induction of labour had burgeoned.[74] Rates of medical intervention have increased further since. Technologies of such kinds can be crucial for optimising the health and well-being of childbearing people and infants, yet as their usage has spiralled over recent decades, often without evidence of benefits for adults or babies, childbearing people are often left feeling frustrated. In a large 2017 study of people who had recently given birth in the US, three-quarters shared the view that obstetric technologies should not be used except when medically necessary.[75] Under 5 per cent of survey participants actually gave birth *without* procedures such as caesarean section, forceps, ventouse, induction of labour, or epidural analgesia.[76] Notwithstanding such dynamics, the systematic *under*-availability of safe obstetric technologies for people who need them, still contributes to unnecessary deaths and mortality across the world, including in so-called 'advanced capitalist' countries.

A key presupposition underpinning Chapter 3 is that obstetric technologies are neither inherently 'good' nor 'bad' – nor do they constitute an homogenous entity. The effects of tools vary considerably, depending upon factors such as how they are used, when, why and for whom. That said, debates around childbirth at times presuppose medical technology to be *either* an intrinsic good *or* an axiomatically detrimental incursion on a time-honoured, physiological process. Ironically, it might be argued that both approaches attribute considerable significance to technology: technology is seemingly constituted as either the *saviour* or the *enemy* of contemporary birthing. In this chapter, I am interested in the power and traction – love it or loathe it – that technology appears to assume within birthing spaces. In order to explore this, I take an analytical dive into and through particular birthing technologies, in order to demonstrate a range of (largely unseen) historical forces, social relations and circumstances which have historically, or in the current era, informed their usage. In addition to important concerns around health and well-being, a range of wider determinants come into play. These include gendered and racialised divisions of labour regulating who can (and can't) use particular technologies; hospital management (not to mention shareholder) concerns regarding staff productivity; the centrality of profit-motives across a range of institutions; public-sector spending cuts, and the financial viability, or otherwise, of birth services in specific geographic and demographic areas. By bringing such dynamics to the foreground of consideration, the role of capitalism in shaping contemporary birthing *through* birthing technologies, can begin to be discerned.

Risk is the focus of Chapter 4. As the influence of medical technologies in pregnancy has burgeoned, references to risk have proliferated too. Use of medical technologies is often legitimised and authorised on the grounds that usage reduces risks of various kinds. Few, if any, obstetric tools are not associated with risk *increases* in specific directions: side-effects, adverse reactions, etc. Childbirth has long been associated with danger, yet the designation of all pregnancies in terms of 'risk' was a twentieth-century development. Even the healthiest of pregnancies are now described in terms of risk – as 'low risk' – within health services. In Chapter 4, the contemporary omnipresence of risk in pregnancy is historically situated with reference to the shifting contours of twentieth-century capitalism. Implicated are concerns over the reproduction of the labour force, the intensification of labour's subsumption under capital, the shift of workers in advanced capitalist countries into intellectual labour, the power of financial capital via such mechanisms as commercial insurance, and harshly changing living conditions. Never before have so many aspects of childbearing been designated as risky. Yet designations of risk do not axiomatically make healthcare safer.

The very idea that healthcare practice should be based upon clear evidence to prove it works and has the desired effects, was hard earned and slow in arriving – particularly in maternity care. Evidence of the RCT variety is the focus of Chapter 5. Scottish doctor, Archie Cochrane, is often considered the trailblazer of the evidence-based medicine movement, and he was an ardent proponent of RCTs. This advocacy was partly based upon his experience of being a prisoner of war during the Second World War. In one of the camps, many of the prisoners had tuberculosis and although there were various medical practices Cochrane could perform to try to help them, he did not know which to use, in what circumstances, or if they were effective.[77] There simply wasn't evidence to support what he was doing. Years later, Cochrane came to view RCTs as crucial for evaluating the effects of medical practices, and he was particularly critical of obstetrics for not developing such studies. Towards the end of the 1970s, he went so far as to describe obstetrics and gynaecology as worthy of a 'wooden spoon' award for failing to scientifically evaluate its own practices.[78] He held the specialty to account for calling healthy women into hospital to give birth and for introducing a range of 'expensive innovations into the routines of pre and postnatal care and delivery' *in the absence of* 'any rigorous evaluation'.[79] Cochrane saw obstetrics as having 'reached its apogee in 1976 when they produced 20 per cent fewer babies at 20 per cent more cost.'[80] Since Cochrane spoke those words, the use of RCTs in relation to birth care has risen exponentially. Medical journals regularly feature the results of Randomised Controlled Trials, and there is a perpetual flow of experiments of this kind being designed and conducted. RCTs are important in birth care, but they are not an historically neutral tool. The reification of RCTs as evidence of best research practice within healthcare can be read as the consolidated effect of various political-economic dynamics integral to capitalism's expansion into the twenty-first century. Moreover, the implementation of RCT findings in relation to birth care is both patchy and wrought with contradiction. These dynamics are explored in Chapter 5.

Given the evidence, risks and technologies which inform contemporary pregnancies, there are today seemingly endless *choices* for people to make whilst gestating. Decisions emerge around which drugs are to be taken, which technologies to opt for, which foods to eat, where to give birth, etc. Choice is the focus of Chapter 6. There is a strong argument that an 'inescapable burden of choice' now characterises contemporary pregnancies, and in that context, questions emerge regarding the extent to which choice is choice at all.[81] Yet it would be naïve to assume that burdens of 'choice' are equitably dispersed across populations. Who gets to choose, how, what and if at all, are key questions which meld into Chapter 6. Such considerations are hued by the many renditions of choice which compete across maternity service contexts. Choice is an ideological tool of neoliberal capitalism, yet whether consumer choice, informed choice, women's choice, or indeed *any* choice is feasible in given situations, indicates the precise ways in which social dynamics have consolidated for different social groups at particular points in time and place.

Given the profound intimacies of childbearing, there are no formulaic approaches that can adequately articulate what needs to be said and done through the spaces of birth across the world. Birth 'care' can be intensely traumatic and unsafe if it does not support, or emerge from, the specific needs of the people who are giving birth and the communities to which they are integral. In the final chapter of the book, I therefore highlight a range of social movements and campaigns through which people are currently working in different areas to improve the conditions in which people birth. Given the expansive impress of capitalism upon contemporary birthing spaces, scope is considered for interconnections and solidarity to be traced and expanded between birth workers, childbirth activists and anti-capitalist endeavours.

Solidarity is at its most powerful when *not* understood as or reduced to a predetermined 'thing' or 'object'. Solidarity is made and formed in the process of struggle. Whereas Marxists have often viewed factory workers and relations between them as key to social change, birth workers and activists across the world have skills and knowledge in relationship building which I contend are crucial for building futures in which exploitation and oppression, and therefore capitalism, are rejected. These are precisely the skills that many birth workers find themselves no longer able to practice within current employment conditions, thereby exacerbating their feelings of alienation and pushing some to leave the healthcare workforce altogether. For instance, the emphasis upon being *with* people that has long been integral to much midwifery practice, may provide a metaphorical touchstone for some of us as we engage in political struggles pertaining to birthing and aspire towards normatively improved futures. The word 'midwife' derives from medieval English where *mid* meant 'with' (and *wif* broadly translated as 'woman'). Being *with* in this sense does not imply presupposing the terms of another person or their labour, but of travelling alongside them, supporting, listening to and responding to what is required. Practices such as these – there are many others – could yet prove crucial in supporting the birthing and nurturing of futures, as well as people, that may yet become possible.

REFLECTIONS ON LANGUAGE

Language is intensely political and through this book I have tried to use words carefully. This is particularly the case in relation to the gender of childbearing people. Through the chapters which follow, I have used a variety of common nouns to signify people who give birth, including 'pregnant person' and 'woman'. However 'natural' the word 'woman' may appear to be as a descriptor of the people who give birth, it is inadequate to signify everybody who bears children. Trans men and gender non-binary people are amongst those who experience pregnancy and childbirth, and it should not be presupposed that gender diversity within the birthing population is a new development.[82] There is little in the way of statistics to ascertain the numbers of pregnant people who are transgender men or who identify outside of the gender-binary. Yet there are no means of acquiring such figures if 'woman' is the only gender category used to describe, and therefore record or count, birthing people.

Gendered common nouns are important for understanding childbirth and this is not least the case when considering historical contexts. The officials who draw up legal and regulatory documents have often used prevailing gender classifications of their time to delineate and define the role of particular groups of people in relation to birth. *The Midwives Act* which passed through the UK parliament in 1902 and which is discussed in more detail in the next chapter, stated that after a specific date 'no woman shall habitually and for gain attend women in childbirth otherwise than under the direction of a qualified medical practitioner, unless she be certified under this Act.'[83] Legislative use of the term 'woman' is significant in this respect, indicating and prescribing highly gendered (not to mention hierarchical) divisions of labour. Yet as Holly Lewis observes, it may be possible to know which categories of gender prevailed during a particular historical period, but that is not the same as knowing who filled those categories or 'which bodies were, empirically speaking, assigned to those categories'.[84] It is not necessarily the case that in early twentieth-century England, all midwives, even if classified as women, were female as that might today be defined. Not all doctors, even in an era in which doctors were categorised as men, were raised as boys.[85]

Gender categories are also significant in contemporary birthing spaces and again Holly Lewis' analysis is useful when considering this. Lewis observes that 'female-assigned persons pressured into womanhood and heteronormative arrangements' constitute a large proportion of the people living across the world today.[86] Here, the word 'pressured' does not necessarily mean that people are forced against their will to live according to particular understandings of 'womanhood', although they may be. The word indicates that specific gender formations, social (including familial) structures and ideological configurations are highly normalised. Marxist-feminists have written on the dynamics of gendered relationships integral to capitalism, and aspects of their analyses are discussed in the next chapter. For the time being, suffice to say that given the oppressive nature of such relations and social forces, I understand why many commentators on birth care have sought to encourage and affirm the power and authority of women when giving birth. But oppression assumes many forms in the context of childbearing, with racism, colonialism, ableism, hetero- and cisnormativity being highly prevalent. That needs to be acknowledged in the language we use around childbirth.

Marxists have also acknowledged sex, in addition to gender, as socially constituted.[87] They are not alone in so doing. At times these writers have drawn upon the scholarship of gender theorist Judith Butler in their analyses. In the words of Rachel Aldred, 'Judith Butler is not a Marxist, but many of her concerns are ours too.'[88] For Butler, sex is a categorisation that operates with violence and force in the world, as does the 'discursive ordering and production of bodies' in accordance with that category.[89] Contemporary midwives, doctors and nurses are expected to assign the sex of a baby at birth, and for those infants identified as intersex (definitions of intersex vary considerably), medicalisation and surgical intervention is often instigated before the child is of an age to consent. As designations of intersex vary, it is hardly surprising that so too do those of sex. 'What *is* "sex" anyway?' enquires Butler.[90] Understandings of sex which prevailed in the era of Marx and Engels, would have been based largely upon the way that genitals appeared to people. By the end of the twentieth century, Butler was able to ask of sex: 'Is it natural, anatomical, chromosomal, or hormonal ... ?'[91] The sexing of bodies is also bound with intensely social presuppositions. These include assumptions that females can, by definition, gestate. Yet not all can, and not all do. In capitalism, the workers deemed most likely to have babies ('females') are often perceived to be a less reliable long-term investment in the workforce than are other workers, and in general their wages are lower.[92] This is the case whether or not these people *actually can or will* get pregnant, have children, or leave the workplace to care for children. In short, being 'female' is not a neutral biological fact: it is infused with intensely social meanings. As people who give birth are very often assumed to be female, it is important to bear in mind the limitations of such codifications.

For reasons mentioned in the above paragraphs, I have used a range of words – some overtly gendered and others not – in reference to people who give birth. At times, my decisions around terminology have depended upon context, and at various points, I have attempted to reflect the language of another writer or researcher whose ideas or calculations I am seeking to portray. Some theoretical arguments can hardly, if at all, be adequately conveyed without the use of specific terminology. Activists and scholars who are committed to writing about reproduction in inclusive ways and who draw upon a range of discursive strategies to do so, have acknowledged inconsistencies and/or imperfections in their use of language.[93] In 2019, George Parker wrote that 'By using a diversity of language forms I am signalling the current limitations of language to describe the diversity of gender in relation to reproductive experience.'[94] My own approach to the use of words in this book is also informed by acknowledgement of the shortfalls of language in relation to human diversity. In addition to that, decisions I have made around the use of discursive forms have been influenced by the geographical scope of the book. For instance, if this book were focused entirely on pregnancy and childbirth in Aotearoa New Zealand, I anticipate that I would have used the word whānau far more frequently than I have. Whānau broadly translates from te reo Māori into the English language as extended family, although the word has more expansive meaning than such a translation suggests.[95] In midwifery care, the word whānau incorporates the childbearing person within the context of their family, friends and/or wider networks of support people who are important to them.[96] The word whānau is also gender neutral. Although I occasionally use the word whānau in the chapters that follow – and in my everyday research and teaching work in Aotearoa New Zealand that focus is important – this book considers birth in a range of lands in addition to Aotearoa New Zealand. In those wider countries the word whānau is not part of the local languages. For that reason, I do not use the word whānau in relation to contexts which include birth beyond Aotearoa New Zealand.

In using a range of discursive mechanisms to describe people who bear children, I have attempted to write this book in a way that aspires towards futures where oppressions, of gendered and other varieties, have ceased to operate. That said, language and the use of language is not static. If I were to write another book on childbirth in a few years' time, I anticipate that the words I might use and the repertoire of terminology available, would be different from those which appear through the pages of this text. In the chapters that follow, some of the issues mentioned in this section are touched upon in more detail, drawing more specifically upon literature which situates gender and birth in the context of Marxist political economy.

2
Stretch Marx

It is seldom recognised that Marx acknowledged human procreation as playing an important role in relation to human history. In 1846, he wrote, with his co-writer Friedrich Engels, that people 'must be in a position to live in order to be able to "make history"', and together they identified the 'production of life' (including the generation 'of fresh life in procreation') as integral to that.[1] That 'people propagate their kind' was seen by them as one of the few dimensions of social life to have endured since time began.[2] To not many aspects of social existence did Marx and Engels attribute such enduring material gravitas across generations, eras and geographical locations. One was that people act in order to meet basic survival needs such as eating and staying warm. Another was that the satisfaction of such needs gives rise to the emergence of new needs. Together they considered these three elements, or 'moments', as asserting themselves throughout history, with the present being no exception.[3] Soon after Marx's death, Engels wrote the following:

> According to the materialistic conception, the determining factor in history is, in the final instance, the production and reproduction of immediate life. This, again, is of a twofold character: on the one side, the production of the means of existence, of food, clothing and shelter and the tools necessary for that production; on the other side, the production of human beings themselves, the propagation of the species.[4]

It is debatable whether Marx would have agreed. When Marx and Engels were writing together, they included the making of people as integral to human history, but they did not emphasise this production of persons as determinant in historical terms. Instead they argued that human history must always be considered in relation to the operations and development of industry and of the exchange of goods.[5]

Marx has been held to account for failing to adequately consider people production within his work.[6] Many of Marx's own references to pregnancy and childbirth were certainly metaphorical in kind. He emphasised, for instance, that the social relationships of a new society 'never appear before the material conditions of their existence have matured in the womb of the old society'.[7] He wrote that 'any old society which is pregnant with a new one' needs a 'midwife' to facilitate the transition.[8] There was certainly historical, if not analytic, logic to his apparent oversight. At the time he was writing, the world was grappling with the effects of a rapidly expanding set of political-economic relations that were spurring unprecedented change in virtually all areas of life. Particularly in his later works, Marx was intent upon analysing that newly emergent, burgeoning, network of aspects and relations. If Marx did not *prioritise* the making of people – particularly in his analysis of capital – perhaps that is precisely because capital did not prioritise, nor have a structural obligation to care for, the making of people. As will be apparent through this chapter, his references to childbirth often relate to precisely this fact.

Notwithstanding that, it's also important to remember that Marx and his co-writer Engels 'were still a couple of bourgeois men in the nineteenth century'.[9] They were also European, and childbearing is far from the only subject matter that they did not substantially theorise in their analyses of capitalism. The revolutionary psychiatrist from Martinique, Frantz Fanon, argued that the ideas of Marx must be expanded upon when colonial contexts are being considered. In colonised countries, the people who rule are distinguished by 'neither the act of owning factories, nor estates, nor a bank balance', although they may have all of these.[10] Those who assume power are 'first and foremost those who come from elsewhere'.[11] He saw that 'Marxist analysis should always be slightly stretched' when considering colonial oppression and rule.[12] There are indeed long and radical traditions which draw upon, whilst stretching, the work of Marx.[13] In such ways, people, histories and dynamics of exploitation and oppression, that were not centred in Marx's critique of capital, are brought to the foreground of consideration. For instance, Fanon himself wrote of the prevalence of psychological trauma, and more specifically '*puerperal psychosis*', amongst childbearing women who were refugees on the Moroccan and Tunisian borders during the Algerian war of independence.[14]

Taking inspiration from the motif of 'stretch Marx', this chapter draws together ways in which Marx, and others in the broad historical materialist tradition, have referred to pregnancy and childbirth in their work. Particular consideration is given to how generations of Marxist theorists and activists have extended the work of Marx in specific directions. They have often done so by applying his methodological approach to later historical contexts and/or by emphasising the preconditions upon which Marx's own work depended but did not explicate. Focus is given to how gestation and birth are referred to within such texts, and in order to contextualise that, a number of key Marxist concepts are also introduced and explained. Within this chapter occasional non-Marxist texts are drawn upon for such purposes as the provision of supporting factual information.

CAPITAL CARES LITTLE

Marx understood that although capital is decidedly unconcerned about the conditions in which childbearing takes place, capital depends upon childbearing. In a much-debated passage of his magnum opus, he contended that the 'maintenance and reproduction of the working class remains a necessary condition for the reproduction of capital. But the capitalist may safely leave this to the worker's drives for self-preservation and propagation.'[15] Marx has been criticised for here displaying a 'simple naturalism' – for overlooking the social character of the relations and activities which enable future generations of workers to be produced and labourers to turn up at work each day.[16] It is certainly important to acknowledge, as Susan Ferguson and David McNally do, that just 'like procreation, drives for self-preservation and propagation are organised within socio-cultural forms of life.'[17] Yet Marx's words can also be read as a declaration that capitalists are largely unconcerned with how workers reproduce, regenerate and renew themselves, *so long as* the capitalist's own capacities for self-preservation and accumulation remain unthwarted and unthreatened.[18] Indeed, the sentence that immediately followed the above quotation from Marx, began in the following way: 'All the capitalist cares for is to reduce the worker's individual consumption to the necessary minimum … .'[19] However good-willed and pleasant an individual capitalist may be, it is structurally imperative that they keep business costs – not least wages with which workers purchase the necessities for their survival and reproduction – as low as is socially feasible. In this way, capitalists aim to remain competitive in the market, survive as capitalists and, ideally, maximise profits. It is therefore hardly surprising that Marx, but particularly Engels, expressed concern (as discussed in more detail below) about the social conditions in which nineteenth-century working-class women in England gestated, gave birth and/or lactated. In order to contextualise this aspect of their work, a detour via Marx's understanding of the circuit of capital is informative.

For Marx, a capitalist is not somebody who acquires riches by saving and hoarding. Capitalists spend money with the explicit aim of making more money and as they do so, capital changes in the shapes and forms it assumes. They use capital in the form of money to purchase the means of production and labour power; they put the labour power to work (which basically involves workers doing their designated work); extra value (surplus-value) is thereby produced by the workers and because of that, capitalists can sell the end product for more than they initially outlaid. Capitalists will spend some of the money (profit) thereby gained on their personal consumption (probably including luxury items), taxes, etc.[20] If they are to continue as capitalists, they must also invest an amount of the profit in purchasing more labour power and means of production in order that they can carry on in business. In this way, money in the form of capital is invested into the production cycle again. It is converted into labour power and means of production, and the cycle is repeated (again and again). As more money is pumped into the means of production, capital grows. Marx depicted the circuit of capital in the formulaic terms *M–C... P... C'–M'*, where *M* stands for money, *C* for commodity and *P* for production.[21] *C'* and *M'* 'denote an increase in *C* and *M* as the result of surplus-value' produced by the workers, and the 'dots indicate that the circulation process is interrupted' whilst production is in process.[22] *L* is labour power and *mp* is means of production, therefore $C = L + mp$.[23] Capital assumes these various forms (money, means of production, purchased labour power) as it circulates to accumulate.

In capitalism, most commodities are produced *within* the circuit of capital. A primary exception is the commodity that is labour power. To quote Tithi Bhattacharya, 'The production of labor power ... takes place outside the immediate circuit of capital but remains essential for it.'[24] Workers are the bearers of labour power, and the production of future workers (which involves the birthing as well as care of new generations of people who may one day become workers) is simultaneously *distinct from*, yet entwined with, the circuitous movement of capital. Although much of the focus of Marx's work involved activities occurring within the circuit of capital, he did at times write about the production and reproduction of labour power. He often framed such discussions in terms of consumption. Marx observed, for example, that the wages workers receive in return for their labour power are used to purchase items of consumption to enable the survival of workers and their dependents. In his own words, the 'capital given in return for labour-power is converted into means of subsistence which have to be consumed to reproduce the muscles, nerves, bones and brains of existing workers, and to bring new workers into existence.'[25] Whether workers perform activities such as eating, drinking or procreating in their own interests or 'to please the capitalist' is, for Marx, 'something entirely irrelevant to the matter'.[26] Capitalists benefit from such activities, even though responsibility for such processes does not lie with the capitalist class. Generally speaking, the financial costs of these activities on the part of the working class are paid for through workers' wages, or at times through state provision (funded via general taxation and therefore also wages), or even charity. Yet as discussed above, capitalists tend towards keeping the amount that they pay for labour power – and therefore the money that the working class can spend on living and reproducing itself – as low as is socially feasible in order that surplus-value can be maximised. In the absence of protective employment legislation, capitalists are also under no obligation to purchase the labour power of one worker rather than another, although capital investment in labour power needs to continue.

It is within this context that Marx's descriptions of the conditions in which nineteenth-century English workers gestated and gave birth, can be read. He saw that due to low pay and associated highly pressured work conditions, the bodies of workers in Victorian capitalism were being worn out whilst they were still very young. He described 'early marriages' (a euphemism for childbearing at a relatively young age) as 'a necessary consequence' of that.[27] Wages earned by young children were essential to support adults (themselves still relatively young) whose bodies were so worn out they could no longer labour, and in that way, Marx contended that capitalist dynamics of the time facilitated working-class population growth despite high death rates.

Marx was also aware of working-class women giving birth in very poor living conditions. He gave the example of two sisters having 'a child' whilst living in the corridor of a cramped house in Berkshire, and of at least one of them going 'to the workhouse for her confinement' before returning home.[28] In a footnote, he indicates awareness that doctors were attending births in small unventilated homes, where 'they found their feet sinking in the mud of the floor.'[29] Such obstetricians 'were forced (an easy task!) to drill a hole through the wall to effect a little private respiration.'[30]

Engels also wrote of the conditions in which working-class women gestated and gave birth. He described women being unable to take time off work during pregnancy for fear of losing their pay. Factory operatives 'when pregnant, continue to work in the factory up to the hour of the delivery, because otherwise they lose their wages and are made to fear that they may be replaced if they stop away too soon.'[31] He indicated that they were expected to work about 12–13 hours a day up until the very end of pregnancy, continually standing, stooping and bending. It was far from unheard of for women to work so late into pregnancy that they ended up giving birth in the factory: 'the case is none too rare of their being delivered in the factory among the machinery.'[32] Notwithstanding such eventualities, around the time that Marx and Engels were writing, the majority of births took place in the rooms and abodes where people lived. Some workhouses provided maternity care and at times, women deemed insufficiently destitute to live in workhouses were permitted to birth there. 'Lying-in hospitals', funded by donations and philanthropy, had also been developed in various localities. They were often aimed at providing care for some of 'the respectable working poor',[33] defined not least by marital status. Marx and Engels were accurate in depicting the circumstances in which many women gestated and birthed, as harsh.

That capital cared little for the conditions in which workers birthed was also the concern of Alexandra Kollontai, a key figure in the Russian Bolshevik Party. In her depiction of the pregnancy circumstances of a range of women in pre-revolutionary Russia, she contrasted the environments in which 'the factory director's wife' and various working-class women had their babies.[34] Mashenka, the rich woman, was encouraged to eat luxury food during pregnancy, and to rest frequently. On the day of the birth:

> The house is a flurry of doctors, midwives and nurses. The mother lies in a clean, soft bed. There are flowers on the tables. Her husband is by her side; letters and telegrams are delivered. A priest gives thanksgiving prayers. The baby is born healthy and strong. That is not surprising. They have taken such care and made such a fuss of Masha.[35]

By contrast, the laundry worker employed in Mashenka's house washed other people's clothes and carried heavy wet linen throughout her pregnancy. She gave birth to 'a thin little mite' behind a curtain in a crowded room, and laboured whilst trying not to wake others who were working the following day.[36] A midwife was present and left soon afterwards, hurrying 'off to another birth'.[37] A further woman, young and without home or work, gave birth 'under a fence in a suburban backstreet'.[38] 'She enquired at a maternity home, but it was full. She knocked at another but they would not accept her, saying she needed various bits of paper with signatures.'[39] The baby of a dye-worker died before birth: 'The steam the mother inhales at the factory has poisoned the child while it was in the womb.'[40]

Such writers depicted a litany of working conditions and hazards impacting negatively upon pregnancy, growing babies and/or childbirth. There was too much stooping, hurried physical activity 'up and downstairs', 'noxious fumes', infertility, stillbirth,[41] not to mention 'deformities of the pelvis' and 'of the hipbones'.[42] 'That factory operatives undergo more difficult confinement than other women is testified to by several midwives and accoucheurs, and also that they are more liable to miscarriages', wrote Engels.[43] He was also concerned about situations in which women were obliged to return to work immediately after childbirth:

> I once heard a manufacturer ask an overlooker: 'Is so and so not back yet?' 'No.' 'How long since she was confined?' 'A week.' 'She might surely have been back long ago. That one over there only stays three days.' Naturally, fear of being discharged, dread of starvation drives her to the factory in spite of her weakness, in defiance of her pain.[44]

Although precapitalist conditions were far from idyllic, they offered possibilities for life with babies and children that factories and capitalist workplaces did not. Prior to the emergence of capitalism, living and household spaces were sites for a range of activities such as weaving, craftwork and cottage farming, as well as childcare, cooking, etc. With the development of the new mode of production, women were increasingly required, in order to survive and earn money, to work in spaces (such as factories) from which infants were excluded. Susan Ferguson makes the observation that, as capitalism consolidated, not only was the work of making and caring for *people* located 'outside the immediate value circuits of capitalism';[45] there also emerged a spatial separation of activities. Work which focused upon immediately sustaining and supporting human beings was 'generally performed in communities and private households (away from work performed for capitalists)'.[46] In the words of Kollontai, 'When the factory gates slam behind her, a woman has to say farewell to maternity, for the factory has no mercy on the pregnant woman or the young mother.'[47] Engels expressed concern about escalating infant mortality rates in such conditions, specifically in nineteenth-century England:

> That the general mortality among young children must be increased by the employment of the mothers is self-evident, and is placed beyond all doubt by notorious facts. Women often return to the mill three or four days after confinement, leaving the baby, of course; in the dinner-hour

> they must hurry home to feed the child and eat something, and what sort of suckling that can be is also evident.[48]

He cites testimonies of the time, according to which lactating women were working away from their babies for long durations: 'My breasts have given me the most frightful pain, and I have been dripping wet with milk.' '[A]ll day the milk pours from her breasts, so that her clothing drips with it.'[49] Marx too was concerned about high mortality rates amongst infants, which was attributed in large part 'to the employment of the mothers away from their homes'.[50] He wrote of infants being given opiates to calm them whilst their mothers were at work.[51] He spoke of it not being possible to 'entirely suppress' some 'family functions', by which he meant 'nursing and suckling children'; and in that context 'the mothers who have been confiscated by capital must try substitutes of some sort.'[52] Although working-class women had long worked as wet-nurses for the wealthy, it was not long after Marx wrote the first volume of *Capital* that commercial production of infant formula developed into a sizeable capitalist industry.[53]

BIRTHING CAPITALISM: APPROPRIATION BY FORCE

If capital cares so little for the conditions in which people live, gestate and produce new people, questions emerge regarding why workers continue to grease the cogs of capital's circulation by going to work each day. Marx made sense of this by reference to what he calls the 'pre-history of capital'.[54] This pre-history varies from country to country, yet elemental was the severing 'from the soil' of the peasant, the 'agricultural producer', the person who grew food for their kin.[55] For example, in England, land enclosures were enforced on peasants from the medieval era onward. Access to the terrain necessary for small-scale farming and grazing was thereby curtailed, restricted, prohibited. Peasants, liberated from the fetters of feudal society, had no option but to become sellers of their own capacity to work (of their own labour power). In this way, they became the working class, the proletariat.

Marx referred to such severing of the people from the land, and from the means of production more generally, as 'so-called primitive accumulation'. There is variation in his accounts, yet he broadly saw the word 'primitive' as referencing a preliminary stage necessary for the development of capitalism.[56] He was also aware that this violent 'pre-history' is largely erased from mainstream accounts of capital's origins, which instead rely upon mythical assumptions that some people were simply more diligent and frugal than others. Marx saw there to be widespread social amnesia surrounding the violence necessary for the transition to capitalism, and this point has been emphasised through the use of graphic birth imagery. In the words of Terry Eagleton:

> Successful revolutions are those which end up by erasing all traces of themselves. In doing so, they make the situation they struggled to bring about seem entirely natural. In this, they are a bit like childbirth. To operate as "normal" human beings, we have to forget the anguish and terror of our births. Origins are usually traumatic, whether of individuals or political states. Marx reminds us in *Capital* that the modern British state, built on the intensive exploitation of peasants-turned-proletarians, came into existence dripping blood and dirt from every pore.[57]

It is not necessary to accept Eagleton's view of birth as intrinsically traumatic in order to understand the point, that capitalism was founded on violence and the expropriation of land from peoples. For Marx, this was the case not only in England, but across the globe. He understood colonisation and the transatlantic slave trade as integral to such processes whereby people are violently dispossessed.[58] He was acutely aware that the textile industries and cotton mills in England depended not only upon the labour of English workers, but upon cotton grown by enslaved workers on plantations in the Americas.[59]

More recently, feminists influenced by Marxism have developed accounts of 'so called primitive accumulation' which relate more explicitly to childbirth and the roles of women. Crucial here is the premise that whilst capitalists direct their attentions to efficient oversight of paid-labour and commodity exchange, for capital to continue and to therefore circulate the production of new generations of workers must happen 'behind the scenes' so to speak – largely beyond the purview of individual capitalists. To facilitate this, Silvia Federici argues, capitalism required a 'new sexual division of labour': a division in which the work of women and 'women's reproductive function' was naturalised as the production and 'reproduction of the work-force'.[60] Whilst the 'proletarian body' was regulated and mechanised in factories and agricultural industry, the bodies of women were shaped and articulated into a corresponding 'machine for the production of new workers'.[61] This was a violent process, she contends, involving the erosion and destruction of the knowledge women previously held about bodies, fertility and health generally. Federici positions the witch-hunts in Europe particularly during the sixteenth and seventeenth centuries, as a crucial mechanism by which this was achieved. Swathes of peasant women (sometimes seen as the healers, the midwives, the abortionists and the herbalists of pre-capitalist times[62]) were interrogated, burned at the stake or killed in other ways. Charges of witchcraft often focused upon apparently transgressive reproductive practices, and around the same time women's execution for infanticide was not uncommon.[63] Working at the cusp of new life and death, midwives came under 'suspicion'.[64] Some were associated with practices of infanticide and others were called upon as functionaries to police, investigate and regulate births. The path was paved, Federici argues, for women's control around issues of procreation to be broken.

In so far as parturition is concerned, Federici views the marginalisation of midwives as opening the door for doctors to assume the role of veritable 'givers of life'.[65] Communities of women who had previously supported one another to birth were gradually expelled from the space of parturition: 'women', she indicates, were 'reduced to a passive role in child delivery'.[66] It was men, and comparatively affluent men at that, who began to assume authority as the protectors of new life in capitalism. Thus, Federici contends that along with 'colonization and the expropriation of the European peasantry from its land', essential for the establishment and consolidation of capitalism, was 'the persecution of the witches'.[67] She emphasises that this was the case in both Europe and in the so-called 'New World'.[68] For Federici, such processes of 'so-called primitive accumulation' are not confined to the annals of history. Women and their bodies continued to be subjugated in ways which support the accumulation of capital, to the extent that these processes constitute ongoing features of capitalism itself.

The historical precision of Federici's account of the European witch-hunts, and the lines of causality she assumes, have been called into question.[69] Yet her work is important, not least for the powerful way in which Federici insists that the subjugation of women is an ongoing feature of capitalism. Her work has also encouraged, and contributes to, a growing body of historical-materialist research which emphasises a dimension of 'so-called primitive accumulation' which Marx himself neither entirely denied nor (perhaps) sufficiently stressed: that processes of 'so-called primitive accumulation' are not confined to the annals of capitalist pre-history. Violent appropriation and dispossession are permanent, and often intensifying, features of the capitalist landscape.

Indigenous writers and activists who draw significantly upon the work of Marx have certainly emphasised that the appropriation of land and resources was not a purely historical occurrence – and they have, at times, referred to pregnancy and childbearing as they do.[70] For instance, Matt Wynyard emphasises that the appropriation of land from Māori – through such processes as war, confiscation and the forced imposition of individual land-titles – was crucial for the formation of capitalism in Aotearoa, and not least for the development of New Zealand's largest capitalist industry: agriculture.[71] That ruining of common resources continues. He notes that recently, as a result of potentially toxic levels of nitrates (a pollutant from capitalist dairy farming) in water, pregnant people in a particular area of the country have been warned to monitor nitrates in the (bore) water they drink and/or with which they make up infant formula.[72] The poisoning of land and resources through capitalist agriculture is an ongoing form of appropriation, and the effects impact across generations. If one considers, as Māori scholar Simon Barber – whose work also draws upon Marx – does, that within Te Ao Māori whenua is both 'land' and 'placenta',[73] it should not be assumed that the ongoing effects of dispossession can be anywhere near adequately understood through colonial-capitalist ways of knowing and being.

Within the context of the US, scholars and activists influenced by the work of Marx have written of appropriation and racialised violence, also gesturing towards – and at times emphasising – pregnancy and birthing as they do. In his classic text *Black Marxism,* Cedric Robinson observed that situating slavery solely in terms of capitalist *pre-history* is a profound error, and one that Marx was not entirely innocent of perpetuating: 'For more than 300 years slave labour persisted beyond the beginnings of modern capitalism, complementing wage labour, peonage, serfdom, and other methods of labor coercion.'[74] It has been observed that Robinson did not focus notable attention on reproduction,[75] but he *was* aware that historically in slave plantations fertility rates amongst enslaved workers could be incredibly low and infant mortality high due to the conditions in which enslaved people lived.[76] After the transatlantic slave trade was banned and childbearing by enslaved people became the primary means by which the enslaved working population could be replaced, enslaved women who could gestate and birth were required to do so frequently. Angela Davis powerfully explains in the following way:

> During the first half of the nineteenth century, when the industrial demand for cotton led to the obsessive expansion of slavery at a time when the importation of Africans was no longer legal, the 'slaveocracy' demanded of African women that they bear as many children as they were

> biologically capable of bearing. Thus, many women had 14, 15, 16, 17, 18, 19, 20 children. My own grandmother, whose parents were slaves, was one of 13 children.[77]

At the same time as European women were being reified as 'producers, nurturers and rearers of children', enslaved women were therefore being 'valuated in accordance with their role as breeders'.[78] They were simultaneously forced to continually bear children whilst being denied legal rights as mothers. If capital is frequently able to overlook and neglect childbearing – leaving such matters, in the infamous words of Marx, to 'the worker's drives for self-preservation and propagation' – this is not always the case. In slavery within capitalism, workers have been actively coerced to bear children. Moreover, as Cedric Robinson emphasised, even after the abolition of slavery, capitalism grew, expanded and developed in 'essentially racial directions'.[79] In 1949, communist activist Claudia Jones indicated the effects of this on Black women – who still had to endure living and working conditions far worse than those of the white population. 'Little wonder' she wrote, 'that the maternity death rate for Negro women is triple that of white women!'[80] While Cedric Robinson coined the phrase 'racial capitalism', far more recently the term 'reproductive racial capitalism' has been developed in recognition that racial capitalism is also 'predicated on ongoing reproductive extraction, dispossession, and accumulation'.[81]

POPULATION AND BIRTH CONTROL

Generational replenishment is a structural prerequisite for the continuation of capital, but there are also countless instances within capitalism of people being actively deterred or prevented from having babies. This is not least the case for Indigenous, and other racialised, people. Narratives of 'irresponsible childbearing' especially directed towards welfare recipients, have also long been a feature of media and public discourse. In order to contextualise this in more detail, a brief discussion of Marx's notion of the 'reserve army' of labour is informative – if not definitive.[82]

For Marx, the reserve army of labour is a section of the population which sits largely beyond the labour-force requirements of capital, but nonetheless serves a structural role in facilitating accumulation. People within the 'reserve army' are often drawn in and out of low-paid and precarious labour at the beck and call of employers, as the labour requirements of capital wax and wane according to economic conditions. Simultaneously, the very presence of a reserve army serves to structurally suppress the wages of those who are already in paid employment, as the threat of workers being replaced by members of the reserve army thwarts workers' demands and aspirations around pay. Given that unemployment is therefore structurally generated and facilitative of capital accumulation, stigmas associated with the child-bearing of people living in poverty operate as ideological bulwarks of the status quo. They effectively shift blame for the structural requirements of capital onto the pregnancies of working-class people. It is for reasons such as these that during his lifetime, Marx was an ardent critic of English economist Thomas Malthus, who advocated curbs on biological reproduction in order to guard against food and resource scarcity at a population level. Marx saw Malthus as ostensibly locating responsibility for poverty with population growth and the procreative activities of the working class, rather than with capital for rendering a sizeable sector of the working-class 'relatively superfluous': unemployed and living in profound poverty.[83]

When Angela Davis challenged aspects of the twentieth-century campaign for birth control, she drew on related arguments.[84] Decidedly *not* opposing contraception per se, Davis was confronting neo-Malthusian logics and eugenic assumptions as they plagued prevalent strands of the movement. She was concerned that elements within the birth control movement sought to reduce the numbers of children in working-class and Black families, with eugenic intention. Davis argued that when such logic informs the promotion of birth control in relation to Black communities, the 'progressive potential' of the movement has been scourged: discourses supporting the elimination of racialised peoples have taken hold, the 'individual right to *birth control*' being replaced by 'the racist strategy of *population control*'.[85] In Davis' account, later feminists of the abortion rights movement had also been slow to oppose forced sterilisation as it was imposed upon Women of Colour and used 'as a means of eliminating the "unfit" sectors of the population'.[86] Even in 2022, the year that *Roe v. Wade* was overturned in the US Supreme Court and essentially eradicated abortion access for great numbers of people in the US, forced sterilisation remained legal in numerous states.[87]

Elite groups have not been alone in seeking to direct the fertility of specific working-class groups. Neo-Malthusian influences have also informed historical calls for a 'birth-strike'. In the years immediately preceding the First World War, the German Social Democratic Party (SPD) was ridden with internal conflict over whether a birth-strike – a collective refusal to bear children – was an appropriate political strategy for the party and its members to adopt. Jenny Brown, author of the recent book *Birth Strike*, describes the debates of the time involving profound disagreement between Marxists and those in a more neo-Malthusian camp.[88] From the neo-Malthusian perspective, reducing the numbers of working-class people born through a birth-strike would potentially challenge capitalism's capacity to survive. If working-class families had less children, they may also be able to afford better living conditions and the time available for women to participate in study and political activism would be boosted. There were important arguments against such positions. Key Marxist figures were supportive of personal decisions to use contraception, whilst also locating responsibility for poverty firmly with capitalism rather than childbearing. It was noted that a country could have comparatively low birth rates without improvement in the conditions of the working class. It is one thing for individuals to refuse to bear children, but quite another to advocate a birth-strike as political strategy.

CONTROLLING BIRTH: MEDICINE, MIDWIFERY AND THE CAPITALIST STATE

As the socialist working class in Germany were discussing the regulation of childbearing through such mechanisms as a birth-strike, in England and Wales the effects of the capitalist state becoming involved in the regulation of birth – or more precisely, in the regulation of midwives who attend births – were being felt. Historically, there had been ecclesiastical licensing of midwives, but in 1902 the Midwives Act was passed through Parliament making it illegal (except in specific temporary circumstances) for people to use the term *midwife* to describe themselves or advertise their services *unless* they were registered through the state to do so.[89] In Marxist terms, the state is a key feature of capitalism, serving the role of protecting and ensuring the conditions – via mechanisms including judicial, legislative and carceral – in which capitalism can continue and develop. Brooke Heagerty's historical analysis of the 1902 Midwives Act emphasises precisely that, situating – as it does – the new regulatory apparatus instigated by the legislation as integral to 'a broader attempt to shape working-class life and culture to support and further capitalist relations'.[90] This was an era, Heagerty emphasises, in which middle-class and wealthy philanthropists were motivated by bourgeois concerns regarding the squalor, ill health and high maternal and infant mortality rates endured by large sections of the (particularly urban) working class. Underlying such emphasis, she argues, was anxiety that the most impoverished sections of the poor were ill equipped 'either to defend the

Empire or to labour productively for the British economy'.[91] Depictions prevailed of poor women as inadequate mothers, incapable of protecting their babies' health against the ravages of death and disease which plagued the cities, or of raising polite, hardworking, respectful children (in other words, the next generation of dutiful workers or soldiers). Against a background of concern that 'the most debilitated of the working class also appeared to be the most prolific',[92] many working-class women were considered in need of moral tutelage: the kind of tutelage that educated middle-class women might be well-suited to provide if they stepped into influential social roles such as nursing and midwifery. The Midwives Act was one of a raft of measures aimed at achieving that kind of social reform.

The 1902 Act created a regulatory body – the Central Midwives Board – which was to define, and restrict, the parameters of midwifery practice. New training mechanisms were introduced and an extensive apparatus established to regulate midwifery registration. In addition to local levels of regulatory supervision, midwives failing to adhere to the new stipulations were subject to disciplinary hearings before the Central Midwives Board. If found guilty, they could be revoked of their legal capacity to practice midwifery.[93] Some of the regulations were largely supportive of the health of childbearing people and infants: stipulations around antiseptic usage, for example, are likely to have been beneficial. The new regulations also obligated midwives to call a physician in instances where childbearing complications arose.[94] In this respect, the scope of midwifery practice was restricted to that of 'normal' pregnancy and birth, but precisely what constitutes 'normal' is contentious. Many midwives had learned through decades of experience that they could provide safe care, without medical assistance, for some of the births that were now designated as beyond their scope.[95] In instances of childbearing complications, physician referral was required whether or not the childbearing person or their family could afford doctors' fees.[96] Midwives were thereby legally bound to act as direct channels to the market of comparatively well-paid men, and such stipulations substantially changed the lines of accountability within working-class communities. Previously a working-class midwife's responsibility was to the people and families whom she attended in labour, and they were often part of the midwife's own neighbourhood networks. In light of the new legislation, midwives became accountable to what Heagerty calls 'the requirements of the Rules and the middle and upper class hierarchy of the supervisory apparatus'.[97] She explains that following the introduction of the regulatory infrastructure, a key task of the Central Midwives Board was to destroy the bonds of solidarity between poor women, families and their midwives:

> Midwives and the women they attended were known to protect and defend each other's interests and well-being against local authorities and social superiors. Trained and lay midwives alike covered up abortions gone wrong, or falsified official records to protect the family ... When families pleaded with them to delay sending for the doctor whose fee they could not pay, midwives often abided by their wishes. In turn, if their midwife got into trouble with authorities, the women and their families would often write letters of support, collect signatures in the neighbourhood on her behalf or refuse to co-operate with local officials against her ... .[98]

The very composition of the Central Midwives Board went some way towards undermining that solidarity, comprised as it was of representatives of government and of organisations with stakes in the new legislation (including doctors).[99] It seems that the Board was relatively lenient in disciplining midwives with close social and class affiliations to Board members – less so the working-class midwives.[100] Affirmation of moral character was required for a midwife to attain their state registration, and such 'lapses' as having children outside of marriage, 'extramarital affairs' and drinking alcohol (even when not working) were used as grounds for revoking certification.[101] To a large extent, midwives were now required to abide by the new regulations and associated bourgeois morality, or lose their state registration and therefore means of income.

By the second decade of the twentieth century, two organisations were formed aimed at organising working-class midwives, improving their conditions of work and amplifying their voice around the statutory decision-making which affected them: the British Union of Midwives and the National Association of Midwives. The former was declared a trade union and called for state support for birth services on a national basis, so that all women could be attended by a midwife in labour and all midwives could receive a fair income. Neither of these organisations appears to have been particularly long-lived. They were largely unwelcomed by the upper echelons of the midwifery hierarchy, who saw trade unions and rank-and-file organisations as presenting a serious threat to the hard-earned respectability of midwifery as a profession: a reminder of the 'working-class roots' of the trade.[102]

The study of midwifery regulation by sociologist Evan Willis also draws upon the work of Marx.[103] He situates state licensing and regulation of health practitioners within the context of a transition from 'competitive' or 'laissez-faire' capitalism to monopoly capitalism, indicating that as the era of monopoly capitalism emerged – and capital became more concentrated in the hands of large corporations – the state became increasingly involved in facilitating the production of labour power through intervening in areas such as social welfare and health. Writing in the Australian context, Willis notes that around the beginning of the twentieth century 'concern with the quantity and condition of labour power' had become apparent.[104] He situates state regulation of health-related occupations as a mechanism deemed to address that situation, and as a means through which political-economic changes of the time were to be legitimised within and through the health context.[105] As a range of health occupations thereby came to be legally defined and overseen through mechanisms inscribed by the capitalist state, it was the medical profession which was granted – and assumed – a critical role in overseeing and legitimising the newly formalised divisions of healthcare labour. There was, in short, Willis argues, 'class and state patronage of medicine'.[106] The medical profession assumed authority to influence arenas of health-work that were *not* medicine, whilst itself being largely protected from the oversight or direction of other occupations or professions. The argument has relevance beyond the Australian context. Note, for instance, that in England, it was obstetrician Sir Frances Champneys who first chaired the Central Midwives Board (CMB) when it was founded.[107] He had actively supported the passing of the 1902 Midwives Act which introduced that board, and he remained chairman until he passed away nearly three decades later. There was also no space formally allocated for midwives on the CMB – that is, to reiterate, on the board which regulated midwifery – until many years after the board was established.[108]

Willis emphasises that the securing and maintaining of medical dominance within healthcare involved the formalisation of gendered, as well as class-based, divisions of labour. Health occupations over which medicine has assumed most purview have typically been highly feminised, with nursing and midwifery as most prominent examples. The founder of modern nursing, Florence Nightingale, is widely understood to have modelled nursing as subordinate to medicine from the beginning of her career. In Willis' words, during the Crimean War she 'refused to attend patients unless directed by doctors'.[109] In the interpretation of Marxist sociologist of medicine Vicente Navarro, Nightingale 'spoke about the role of the nurse as one of (1) supporting the physician, equivalent to the supportive role of the wife in the family; (2) mothering the patient; and (3) mastering the auxiliaries'.[110] If those were the origins of modern nursing, midwifery was slightly different. Midwives tended to work independently of physicians, and at the beginning of the twentieth century, Australian doctors were afraid of the threat that well-trained midwives might pose to the income they – as doctors – received from attending births. Doctors were also concerned that midwives might make lucrative incursions into treating various diseases that women endured and doctors attended to.[111] By the end of the 1920s, legislation was introduced which effectively designated midwifery as a specialist area of nursing.[112] That change, Willis contends, had 'the effect of subordinating [midwifery] to medicine much more formally than had previously occurred'.[113] In this way, the principal competitor to obstetrics was largely contained, and births were no longer overseen primarily by 'working class women' but by 'middle class men'.[114] The state-sanctioned transition also had the effect of replicating, within the birth-related occupational division of labour, the structure of gendered divisions of labour prevalent within bourgeois nuclear family structures: 'the male-husband-father-doctor [was] directing and controlling the female-wife-mother-nurse in the interests of the child-patient.'[115] Whether or not the interests of the 'patient' or indeed 'child' were paramount is, of course, questionable.

BIRTH AS LABOUR

If midwives, doulas and health practitioners such as nurses and doctors, are aptly described as *working* when they support a person to give birth, questions have also been asked regarding whether the act of childbirth is in itself labour in the sense of work. Marx and Engels acknowledged pregnancy and childbirth as having distinctly social dimensions, yet they did not go so far as to designate either gestation or parturition as *work* in and of themselves. They considered 'physiological' (or 'natural') divisions of labour to be crucial in many historical and social formations, indicating that a person's biophysical characteristics were important in determining the work they perform.[116] People of particular ages or with specific physical strengths might perform tasks of certain kinds. Those who are lactating are likely to perform work which enables them to stay close to infants who are physically dependent upon that for survival. Whilst corporeal childbearing processes would therefore influence the kinds of work and social activity that people do, that is not to say that gestation and lactation are in themselves labour.

Marx and Engels wrote that 'The production of life, both of one's own in labour and of fresh life in procreation ... appears as a double relationship: on the one hand as a natural, on the other as a social relationship.'[117] Here, the production of 'fresh life' is clearly differentiated from the production of a person's own life, and although the former is achieved through procreation, only the latter is described as work and labour. In relation to this formulation, it is pertinent to ask why the ongoing activity involved in maintaining oneself is constituted as work, but the making of other people isn't. In other words, why is the production of food in contexts such as agriculture or factories considered to be work, whilst the production of nutrients for a foetus or via lactation is not?

In an oft-cited section of *Capital*, Marx wrote that human workers use their bodies and their limbs when they labour, yet the deployment of such corporeal elements is insufficient to constitute work for the human species. Noting that spiders make webs in ways that resemble weaving and that bees construct 'honeycomb cells' in ways that 'put many a human architect to shame', Marx differentiated between the work of people and the activities of other animals in the following way:

> ... what distinguishes the worst architect from the best of bees is that the architect builds the cell in his mind before he constructs it in wax. At the end of every labour process, a result emerges which had already been conceived by the worker at the beginning, hence already existed ideally.[118]

Humans have the capacity to engage in abstract planning of their work, and specifically human work involves precisely that: the realisation of deliberate and purposeful objectives. In so much as that was the understanding of labour underpinning much of Marx's work, it goes some way towards explaining why he did not emphasise human childbearing as work. A vast array of processes integral to gestation occur within a pregnant person's body whether or not they are desired or planned. People may be fully aware they are pregnant whilst simultaneously lacking capacity to control key outcomes of their pregnancies in ways which might be highly important to both them and others. Framed slightly differently, the autonomic nervous system (which is not under conscious control) plays a crucial role in many of the physiological changes which occur during pregnancy. In what she described as her unorthodox 'Hegelian-Marxist analysis' of human reproduction, Mary O'Brien contended that notwithstanding similarities between 'mother and architect', the two are also 'quite different'.[119] Yet if the architect has greater capacity to deliberately and materially build the objects of their imagination, there is also a danger that the role people (especially women) have actively played over centuries in altering and directing the course of lactation and of childbearing more generally, is overlooked. That is to say that such processes, and therefore the work women often do, are all too easily conflated entirely with nature.[120]

In addition to considerations regarding whether pregnancy and birth constitute labour in the sense of work, there have also been reflections within Marxism over whether pregnancy and birth constitute a specific kind of work: that is, productive labour for capital. Within the first volume of *Capital*, Marx designated all labour which produces something as productive labour in the general sense that it makes – *it produces* – something.[121] He warned in a footnote of the limitations of such usage of the term, arguing that such a definition of productive labour 'is by no means sufficient to cover the capitalist process of production'.[122] Within capitalism, he contended, productive labour is that which *directly* produces surplus-value for the realisation of capital: 'Since the immediate purpose and the *authentic product* of capitalist production is *surplus-value, labour is only productive,* and an exponent of labour-power is only a *productive worker* if it or he [*sic*] creates *surplus-value* directly.'[123] During the 1970s, particularly in Italy where the social role of women was largely conflated with that of housewife, feminists influenced by the autonomist workers movement began to ascribe housework (and they included pregnancy and childbirth within that) as *productive* for capital. In a definitive article of the movement, Mariarosa Dalla Costa and Selma James argued that 'housework as work is *productive* in the Marxian sense', that is to say in the sense of 'producing surplus-value'.[124] Indicating that pregnancy is also included within that, in the introduction to the pamphlet Selma James also argued that the production of labour power requires 'nine months in the womb'.[125] In developing such arguments, they were not rigidly adhering to Marx's definition of productive labour, but were instead carving, within workers' struggles, a place – a role 'as protagonist' – for those who perform the largely unseen and unappreciated labour of making and maintaining people in the home.[126] Their argument acknowledged the classically Marxist position that the existence of labour power is a condition of possibility for productive labour in the capitalist factory (and therefore for the direct production of surplus-value for capital), but added to that the premise that the work which produces labour power must therefore also be considered productive labour for capital.

In the early 1980s, autonomist feminist Leopoldina Fortunati explored that formulation of pregnancy and birth as productive labour in more depth. Her words are remarkable, not least for the ways in which she directly and unwaveringly applied categories of Marxist political economy – categories that Marx applied to productive factory labour processes within his own analyses – to pregnancy and childbirth. Firstly, she differentiated the production of labour power, which she considered to occur through pregnancy, from labour power's *reproduction* (which for her involved 'already existing labour-powers').[127] She identified the 'raw materials' involved in the production of labour power as 'sperm' and the childbearing person's (she uses the term 'woman's') 'entire body'.[128] As it is through the latter that the work of building a baby in gestation happens, the pregnant person's body constitutes 'raw materials' as well as 'a means of work'; pregnancy ends with the birth of the baby, at which point 'the product, the new labour-power is produced.'[129] Fortunati therefore emphasises that labour power is always 'raw material' because a person arrives in the extra-uterine world already containing 'nine months' of work.

Whether the production of labour power should be categorised as productive labour for capital has been a subject of debate amongst Marxists. There is certainly a danger, particularly apparent within Fortunati's work as sketched above, that the distinction between the production of life and the production of labour power is lost in some autonomist feminist accounts. For many outside of the autonomist tradition, the ongoing activity of making new generations of the working class is acknowledged as *necessary* for capital, but without this rendering such activities productive labour in the sense of them being directly generative of surplus-value. Paddy Quick was decisive on this point, arguing in 1977 that the labour of childbearing is crucial for the continuation of capital but 'does not constitute the direct performance of the surplus labor which is extracted by the ruling class'.[130] For Marx, surplus labour is the work that employees perform which produces value over and above that of their wages (and wages are generally set at the basic level required for workers to consume sufficiently to reproduce themselves and keep turning-up at work). Surplus labour is therefore that which generates surplus-value for the capitalist class. Quick argued that workers who *do not* produce more than they consume in this way are generally of no use to capital because it is the value which a worker produces above the level of their own needs which constitutes surplus-value and accumulates as capital. Workers who produce less than that can even be considered an overt burden for capital *rather than productive* because they consume resources which might otherwise accumulate for the ruling class. In the case of child-bearing, a contradiction thereby emerges: the capitalist class requires the working class to bear children, and that is helpful to the capitalist in the long term, but when a working-class person is in the process of physically birthing a child and in the period which immediately follows, they are at least temporarily hindered from producing surplus-value in the present. Moreover, on average, women spend less time in waged labour than men do, and they receive disproportionately lower wages for the waged labour they *do* perform, in part *because* they are characterised as a less dependable workforce, deemed more likely to leave to have children.[131] Lise Vogel, whose work is a mainstay of the Social Reproduction Theory strand of Marxism, elaborated on Quick's argument, indicating it is in the interests of the ruling class for strategies to be developed which minimise the work required to reproduce the working class whilst simultaneously ensuring that labour power is readily available.[132] Such strategies, she argued, often avail themselves of and benefit from relationships premised upon kinship and sexuality. Typically, she contends, in class societies the biological father and/or his family supports his partner financially during the period around child-bearing.[133] The pregnant women may well be dependent upon that income long after the immediate childbearing period has ended, as the unpaid labour of raising and maintaining families is highly feminised. In contexts such as these, Vogel argues, men assume a form of structurally constituted dominance within working-class families premised upon their enhanced earning capacity, and it is an authority that is in the interests of the ruling class.[134] Arguably therefore, it is precisely because pregnancy and childbirth *do not constitute* productive labour for the capitalist class (precisely because they do not directly make profit for capitalists) that male supremacy is a constitutive feature of capitalism.[135]

Arguments such as those sketched above tend to presuppose heteronormativity in that they foreground the norms of heterosexual relationships and associated binary constructions of gender. There is also a possibility that such arguments imply, potentially at least, that heteronormativity is grounded in political-economic relations. Which is to say, drawing upon the words of Holly Lewis, that political-economy is causal of the '"normativity" in hetero-normativity'.[136] For instance, there is a strong argument that as the nuclear family rose to prominence from the late nineteenth into the twentieth century, gender came to be seen as a particularly 'rigid binary'.[137] In that context, there arose a strict differentiation between activities that were, to use the terminology and argument developed by Endnotes, directly mediated by the market (those which took place in the paid workplace, for instance), and those which were *indirectly* mediated by the market (such as activities which often took place at home). Whilst historically, the latter group of activities could have been performed by wider family members, within nuclear family units premised upon strictly gendered divisions of labour those tasks were ascribed as essentially female activities. The strict binary constitution of gender indicative of the era thereby mapped directly onto the two spheres of activity, one of which was directly and the other indirectly market-mediated. The former was deemed the domain of men (assumed to be male) and the latter was constituted as the arena of women (assumed to be female). Such binary constitutions of gender were not untypical of the era in which either Quick or Vogel were writing in 1970s and '80s. Through the years of neoliberalism which subsequently developed, many tasks women had performed in the home (such as childcare) increasingly entered the marketplace, not least as incomes were suppressed and families tended to require two incomes to survive. Followed by years of austerity politics when public spending was slashed, there were times when such tasks threatened to move into homes again as welfare provisions for childcare, for example, were cut. Through such shifts – in and out of the market – key tasks, Endnotes indicate, have been *denaturalised* as the inevitable destiny of women. Integral to such processes of denaturalisation, it is contended, gender itself has come to be more widely understood as '*an external constraint*': that is to say, a constraint that can be called into question and challenged.[138] Such arguments may help to explain how it is that over the past decade or two, many prevalent assumptions regarding the gender of childbearing people have been challenged and language accommodating of gender diversity is more widely advocated in relation to pregnancy and childbirth than previously. In so far as that is the case, such developments appear intimately related (which is not to say they are reducible) to shifting allocations of labour associated with movement in the configurations of capitalism.

As the twenty-first century rolled out, discussions around whether pregnancy is productive labour also assumed new points of reference integral to a rapidly changing political-economic environment. The emergence of the commercial surrogacy industry was influential in this respect, seen to facilitate new relationships between gestation and capitalistically productive labour. The extent to which paid surrogates produce *value* in capitalist terms is a subject of ongoing reflection and debate. For Sophie Lewis, they decidedly do. In her own words 'when it is performed for clinical firms, the work that commercial surrogates do creates value … . [I]t is the pregnancy itself that creates the value.'[139] Susan Ferguson is not convinced. She enquires as to how it is possible to ascertain the average labour-time socially necessary to produce the end product, when so much of the production is 'an unconscious, biophysical process'.[140] Ferguson is here inferring Marx's premise that the magnitude of the value of a commodity is determined by the quantity of labour-time that is socially necessary for it to be produced.[141] The premise that surrogacy is value-producing labour certainly invites such questions as to whether surrogates are labouring to produce value when they are sleeping.

The debates around surrogacy have also prompted further reflection on whether *non-surrogate* pregnancies and birthing (the focus of this book) constitute labour in sense of work. In response to Sophie Lewis' provocation that pregnancy is 'gestational labour',[142] Susan Ferguson suggests that active biophysical processes integral to pregnancy are not helpfully defined as *work*.[143] She agrees that pregnant people can deliberately influence and attend to such physiological processes, and that these conscious activities may indeed be considered labour: that is, 'important (and hidden) social reproductive labor'.[144] Nonetheless, many aspects of gestation 'do not constitute *labor* … any more than human respiration does.'[145] I also find it more helpful to think of birthing and pregnancy in terms of physiology (and even biochemistry) at times, than I do to conflate all of human reproduction into the category of labour (as in work). Marx argued similarly in relation to the analysis of aspects of political economy. He contended that in some contexts, it is necessary to hold certain presuppositions stable at the start of analysis. These suppositions may 'become fluid in the course of their development', yet he insisted that 'only by holding them fast at the beginning is their development possible without confounding everything.'[146] Marx was writing about wages, and I argue similarly about differentiations between labour (as in work) and childbearing physiology. Through (at times) maintaining analytic distinction between the two, I find that I am able to consider – or study – the actions that people might take to *support* physiological mechanisms to work well ('optimally' is the language that many people use) in childbearing. This is important, and not least because many people continue to die and be injured unnecessarily in childbirth, and whatever can be done to prevent that is important. That said, precisely because physical health *is* intimately related to human actions – and as Engels saw, working and living conditions – the division between physiology and conscious human activity is far from absolute.

'NEW REPRODUCTIVE TECHNOLOGIES', AND LABOUR AGAIN

As twentieth-century capitalism drew to a close, the development of so-called 'new reproductive technologies' was integral to shifting interpretations of who can, and cannot, give birth and raise children. Marxist-feminist Martha Gimenez wrote of the new technologies of conception, such as *in vitro* fertilisation (IVF), in this respect. She situated their emergence within the context of the 'overall development of the productive forces' of capitalism.[147] For Marx, the productive forces involve a combination of the capacities of labour with means of production, such as technologies and raw materials. Integral to the forces of production is therefore the state of science and knowledge within a given society. The productive forces were seen by Marx to develop and change rapidly in capitalism, due to capital's drive to push technological expansion in the facilitation of capital accumulation. Although Gimenez saw the new reproductive technologies as becoming possible as an effect of the development of the productive forces, she also saw them as holding the potential to facilitate change in the social relations which surround procreation and reproduction. Through the use of such technologies, a range of scenarios become possible in which a person without genetic connections to an infant can gestate and birth that baby. Gimenez thereby identified the potential for a severing of the 'relations of procreation' (human relations that are linked to biological capacity) from the 'social relations of reproduction' (which she saw had tended to be structured according to heterosexual norms including marriage).[148] Firmly entrenched biologically oriented understandings of what it means to be a mother were in the process of being challenged, and such shifts were inseparable from the broader social relations and forces of capitalism. Also writing in the 1990s when technologies such as IVF were new on the market, Angela Davis' analysis had a different emphasis.[149] She was acutely aware that for many women, the fact of bearing a child has not historically guaranteed them rights to raise that child. She was also concerned that the very presence of the new technologies would reinforce (for those with access to them) expectations of a child of 'one's own', whilst many mothers, including Black teenagers, would continue to be stigmatised for birthing babies.

Much has changed since the end decade of the twentieth century. Given the pressures of contemporary capitalism, many can afford neither the time nor money to birth and raise a child. Birth rates are declining as the average age of childbearing is rising. It has been argued that a particular form of 'birth-strike' is taking place, as people refrain from childbearing, not least in the US.[150] A growing range of reproductive technologies have also become available on the market, and a few years ago major companies started to contribute towards the financial costs of egg (oocyte) freezing for members of their female workforce.[151] Whilst some may welcome the opportunity to pause any possibility of growing and birthing babies, Nancy Fraser suggests that such developments are also tantamount to employers saying to their employees: 'wait and have your kids in your forties, fifties, or even sixties; devote your high-energy, productive years to us.'[152] Eggs can also be frozen to be later used in surrogate pregnancies. In this way, a range of reproductive technologies are used to not only delay childbearing, but to transfer pregnancy and childbirth to another person at a future date – often for a financial price. As gestational surrogates are frequently women living in less affluent regions of the world, including the Global South, such practices have been described as resonating with the ideological premises and racial configurations of European colonial history and imperialism of the Euro-American kind.[153] Rather than outright opposition to commercial surrogacy, one suggestion has been to support the self-organising of those who carry out such work, in order that they can command more of the conditions in which they labour.[154]

Such discussions also invite further reflection on the question of whether paid surrogacy is value-producing labour. Whilst for Sophie Lewis it definitely is (as discussed above), Kevin Floyd expressed concern that assertions of commercial surrogacy as value producing fail to sufficiently emphasise the violence of capital in the current era.[155] Drawing upon Marx's understanding that as capital accumulates in its constant form (as physical infrastructure, machinery, labour-saving technologies, devices, etc.), the relative amount of labour power required by capital decreases such that the reserve army of labour grows in relation to the employed population. As capital expansion through the use of labour power has slowed over recent decades, financial services (including those which loan money in return for interest payments) have expanded, and levels of debt have escalated not least for households in the Global South where waged labour is sporadic and very low-paid. In this context, Floyd warns against viewing methods of household income generation such as commercial surrogacy or organ-selling purely in terms of value-producing labour, whilst nonetheless being aware of the dangers of conflating women's bodies with nature. Hence he argues: 'In what may appear an obscene literalisation of the longstanding metaphorics that associate women's bodies with "nature" – in the discourse of ova "harvesting" for example – those bodies are reduced to the status not of living labour but of living raw material.'[156] In so far as commercial surrogacy is concerned, a person's uterus might be considered a means of production rather than raw materials, but the general point Floyd is making remains pertinent. He contends that to refer to such developments as value-producing labour is an ethical intervention – one which upholds respect for women's bodies and activities – but obscures more than it clarifies, and depends upon a somewhat optimistic reading of labour, given the current dynamics of capital.

As the use of 'assisted reproductive technology' has burgeoned, and cord/amniotic stem-cell banking and gamete freezing are normalised, many features of so-called 'biological reproduction' are now extracted, sold, purchased, reconstituted and speculated upon as part of the so-called '*bio-economy*'.[157] A range of hitherto unfeasible developments are beginning to enter the realms of possibility. Uterine (womb) transplantation is an ongoing field of clinical investigation, and in 2023, the first baby outside of a clinical trial was birthed by a woman who had received a uterine transplant.[158] There is medical discussion regarding the feasibility of uterine transplantation pregnancies in transgender women.[159] According to a review of the criteria for uterus transplantation [UTx] in the UK, 'medical barriers to UTx in transgender women and men do not appear to be insurmountable', although it is suggested that there may still be legal or regulatory barriers regarding human embryo transfer in such instances.[160] Complete ectogenesis (gestation entirely outside of the human body) is not yet possible, but may at some point become more than a science-fiction scenario.

Discussions of the ethical, political and scientific dimensions of human ectogenesis are ongoing, and writers influenced by Marxism have not been absent from such debates. Lewis considers ectogenesis as potentially having a role to play in resisting heteronormative nuclear family arrangements:

> I would love to one day see the queer gestational commune in which 'bio-bags' of some kind [for growing foetuses] enabled gestators to pause, share, transfer, redistribute, and walk away from pregnancies. I would love to see these technologies help denaturalize motherhood and liberate those with uteruses from the imperative to gestate.[161]

She suggests that for technologies to be developed and used in ways such as this, they would need to taken out of the hands of an elite capitalist class. Her text resonates with aspirations expounded by Shulamith Firestone in the 1970s. In her classic text *The Dialectic of Sex*, Firestone commended the analysis of Marx and Engels but considered that it did 'not go deep enough'.[162] Her own vision of a vastly improved society required '*freeing … women from the tyranny of reproduction by every means possible*'.[163] To this end, she advocated taking so-called 'biological reproduction' entirely outside of the human body. Her argument resonates with contemporary calls for 'full-automation' or 'luxury communism', according to which work is eradicated in a post-capitalist society through the deployment and development of advanced technologies.[164]

The extent to which it would be emancipatory to entirely mechanise pregnancy and birth is of course controversial. Underpinning such utopian aspirations tend to be assumptions that pregnancy and childbirth are, to invoke Firestone's terminology, *tyrannical* in some way. Lewis writes of being fascinated by 'pregnancy's morbidity'.[165] There is undoubtedly death in birth, and parturition can be experienced in intensely traumatic ways. Given the profoundly social determinants of that, I may be less inclined than many to attribute blame to childbirth itself – as if birthing is ever unshaped by the societies in and to which 'it' is a contributing process. Federici expresses concern that ectogenesis would enable planning of precisely the populations required for capitalism to function most efficiently: people who are more complicit and 'robot-like' than we appear even today.[166] If such technologies were to become a reality, and sold to us as liberation, it is also difficult to see how gestation and childbirth could be entirely eliminated without considerable coercion and force. Many people – cisgender, transgender and non-binary – *do* want to gestate and give birth. There is no longer (if there ever was) a legitimate vantage point from which it might be assumed that they have simply been duped. There are also long histories – racist, ableist, eugenic – of forced abortion and sterilisation. In this regard, there is an intensely political need to stick with pregnancy and childbirth; and to take the shifting shapes and parameters of those 'moments' seriously.

TAKING STOCK

As demonstrated in this chapter, Marx and those who have developed and expanded upon the corpus of his ideas, have referred to pregnancy and childbirth in many different ways. Gestation and birthing have been referred to as natural, social, labour and work. They are seen as activities that have persisted since the beginning of human history; processes that are needed by capital, but not supported by capital. They are activities forced upon enslaved people, and capacities associated with specific 'types' of bodies. Gestation and childbearing are to be encouraged, prevented, avoided, delayed, or paid for. They are blamed for working-class poverty, regulated by state mechanisms and controlled by men in white coats. They used to be understood by women who were burned at the stake. They are tyrannical. Or not. They are to be taken out of the human body. They are here to stay. In the afterword to his book *The Limits to Capital*, David Harvey described 'the birth of a working-class child' as 'a simple event'.[167] More precisely, he was of the view that if Marxists are to study and understand how labour power is reproduced within and through the lived experiences of working-class people, the starting point for analysis must be very different from that with which Marx began his analysis of capital. Marx started his analysis of capital with the commodity – the individual commodity – and from there he interrogated and traced the relations and dynamics which enable the commodity to manifest as the basic form of wealth within capitalism. In order to study labour power's reproduction, Harvey argues, it is necessary to start from the moment of a person's birth and to take account of the socialisation and related process which follow. In many ways, Harvey was not wrong to describe 'the birth of a working-class child' as a 'simple event'. It may appear precisely that way within a person's life trajectory: a basic point of departure from which the rest of their life unfolds. But if we explore and investigate the 'moment' that is childbirth with curiosity and intrigue, it is not difficult to identify many interactions and determinants that come together in birthing and that shape and ascribe its parameters. Birth is not 'just' the starting point of a person's extra-uterine life, but a 'moment' in and through which a vast range of intensely social, as well as physiological, dynamics coalesce.

Perhaps it is not surprising therefore, that childbirth has been considered a site of potential social transformation. In her introduction to an edited collection of narratives of birth workers such as midwives and doulas, published in 2016, Silvia Federici reflected that the building of alternative societies begins with change at the level of the activities and relationships through which people restore and rejuvenate themselves and one another, and live their everyday lives.[168] She described birth work as 'paradigmatic' in this respect. Such work is an intensely political undertaking through which people are supported – at a time in their lives often associated with exposure and vulnerability – to be autonomous, strong and to start on journeys of 'self-valorization'. For Marx, valorisation is the process through which capital reproduces and grows due to the value-producing labour of workers. Self-valorisation of the most exploited and oppressed groups therefore involves people growing, building and augmenting *themselves*, independent of the parasitic life-sucking draws of capital and its associated institutions. I find the idealism of Federici's text inspirational, whilst at the same time a little unsettling. Birthing can certainly be transformational, and in many ways. Some of these ways are incredibly life-affirming for people generally, as well as women. Others are intensely traumatic. Parturition can be supported in ways that instil confidence and trust in a birthing person's ability to move and act in the world in ways that matter. Birthing can be a powerful collective event, through which communities who will support and raise a child together, move into their newly emergent roles and jointly usher in the new life with and alongside which they will all grow. I entirely support those birth workers who act to make that a reality for people. If capital self-valorises because labour creates value, the autonomy of capital is never absolute, and therefore resistance and activity which aims to meet community needs is possible. *But* – and this is where my hesitancy comes in – birth workers are also overworked, exhausted, underpaid, burnt-out and feel unable to do the work they *really* want to do, and they are so precisely *because* of capital. By my reading, there is as yet little Marxist analysis which has sought to grapple with and understand in depth the conditions in which contemporary birth workers such as midwives, doulas, nurses, etc. labour, and in which people therefore birth. (The studies of Willis and Heagerty make insights which retain relevance today, but they are historically focused.) The development of such analyses is important and necessary if we are to understand why and how it is that birth work is currently under the constraints that it is, and to develop the most effective and durable strategies for transformation.

The funding and ownership of birth services are crucial considerations in this respect. It might be assumed that for perinatal services to be capitalist, they must be privately owned, profit-making businesses. Some certainly are, but far from all. Within capitalism, pregnancy and birth services can be owned and funded in many different ways. These services can be state-owned institutions funded via general taxation. Some are commercial enterprises or supported through charity donations. Birth care can be paid for from private sources including the wages of childbearing people, private health insurance and/or a mixture of both. In the UK and Aotearoa New Zealand, most birth care is state-funded and free at the point of access, although private services also operate and sometimes do so within public hospitals. In the US, birth care tends to be paid for through health insurance which can be purchased by individuals or their employers, as well as there being state insurance programmes such as Medicaid. The funding arrangements of pregnancy and birthing services are complex, and they *do* – or at least can – make a difference to the care that is provided. Yet capitalism influences healthcare in ways which extend well beyond funding arrangements and revenue streams, and birthing services (despite the diversity of their operational arrangements) share many characteristics in common. That is where the TREC quartet – technology, risk, evidence and choice – is important. Through starting with these 'concrete' features of birthing spaces, it is possible to trace the ways in which capital caresses and shapes what happens within those environments, often 'behind the back' of those working and birthing there. I begin that tracing with an exploration of obstetric technology.

3
Technological Fetish in the Birth Chamber

The use of obstetric technologies has risen rapidly over recent decades. In the United States, the caesarean section rate was 5.5 per cent in 1970, 16.5 per cent a decade later, and had risen to 32 per cent by 2017.[1] Around a third of people who gave birth in England in 2011–12 either had their labour induced *or* had a caesarean section before they went into labour; ten years later, the equivalent figure had risen to 53 per cent.[2] In Aotearoa New Zealand, the 2021 caesarean section rate was 30.9 per cent, and rising too over the preceding few years had been rates of induction of labour, episiotomies and epidurals.[3] The proliferating use of medical technologies might not be problematic if health benefits accrued similarly, or if childbearing people were actively pushing for such spiralling levels of technological intervention. There is little evidence to suggest that either is the case. For instance, notwithstanding increasing rates of various interventions, the latest data on the UK context indicates that the maternal death rate has actually been rising (even when COVID-related deaths are taken out of the equation), and rates of stillbirth reduction are described as stagnating.[4] There are certainly circumstances in which staff failure to use a particular technology has harmful effects, and women also actively request a range of technologies including pharmacological pain relief. Yet research carried out in advanced capitalist countries demonstrates that many childbearing people would prefer to have less medicalised birth experiences than they actually do.[5] The emphasis of this chapter is that the deployment of obstetric technologies in birth is prompted by far more than concern for the well-being of pregnant childbearing people and babies. An experienced UK midwife speaks of birth workers being increasingly caught up in 'a real fear of not using all the technology available'.[6] Doctors have internationally declared escalating caesarean section rates to be beyond the collective control of themselves as physicians.[7] In short, it would appear that machines and technologies, rather than people, have become the guiding force – 'the virtuoso', to use Marx's terminology[8] – of many birthing environments. That is the focus of this chapter.

The word 'technology' derives from the Greek language: *technê* refers to art and craft, and *logos* signifies words.[9] When the term 'technology' first became part of the English language, it was used in reference to discussion (words) within the arena of the applied arts – which is to say, bodies of knowledge regarding the way the world is changed through the deliberate articulations and crafting of human beings. Today the word has different connotations, and not least within birthing arenas. In this chapter, the word 'technology' is used in two interrelated ways, both of which correspond with contemporary usage of the word in hospitals and birth service contexts. Firstly, I use the word in reference to material objects and physical tools – such as devices, machines, pharmaceuticals, etc. – which are integral to the work process of nurses, midwives and doctors. Secondly, I used the word to denote clinical practices which involve the use of a range of these other technologies and are also integral to the labour processes of paid birth workers. A caesarean section would fall into this latter category, as involved are sterile surgical instruments, pharmaceuticals, infusion pumps for delivering pharmaceuticals, drip-stands, monitoring machines, obstetric gel, suture materials, specialist lighting, etc. During childbirth, a range of technologies can certainly be used and deployed by childbearing people and their loved ones, rather than by paid birth workers. These are gestured towards at times in the analysis that follows. However, when the use of birthing technologies is discussed in medical (or wider) journals, evaluated in clinical trials, or quantified in national-level statistics, it is overwhelmingly technologies which are constitutive components of the labour process of *clinicians*, that are being referred to. For that reason, these are the focus of this chapter.

Over the pages that follow, attention is given to the social relations, forces and elements integral to capitalism which have supported obstetric tools to gain such import and traction within birthing arenas. I begin with consideration of some of the earliest technologies of modern obstetrics, particularly forceps and then twilight sleep. This is followed by a brief foray into Marxist theory which supports consideration of technology as fetish (as an incredibly alluring, beguiling force enlivened by intricate unseen networks of social relations) and of some of Marx's reflections on technology as capital. These insights inform the discussion of two more contemporary obstetric practices: the 'active management of labour' (an amalgamation of technologies which came to prominence during the latter decades of the twentieth century) and caesarean section. Yet one of the problems which haunts contemporary capitalism is that whilst technologies are vastly overused, there are also 'deserts' within which contemporary technologies of birth are much needed or wanted but not available. I end the chapter with consideration of that issue.

LOCAL CONSOLIDATIONS OF GLOBAL HISTORY

Technologies of parturition long pre-date the birth of capitalism. For millennia, people have used and developed an array of tools to assist in childbirth: from herbal remedies, to specially designed stools, bricks for squatting on during labour and doubtless far more. Caesareans have been conducted since ancient times, at least to save the life of a baby.[10] In early modernity, oils, lubricants and enema syringes were used by midwives.[11] Yet it is forceps which are considered the signature tools of early modern obstetrics.

The development of these blades in seventeenth-century Europe made it possible for women and babies to survive cases of very difficult labour, where previously at least one of them would have lost their life.[12] The Chamberlen family of barber surgeons and obstetricians, who were known for attending members of the nobility and royal family in childbirth, are attributed with the invention of forceps. They also guarded the secret of their new technology for around a century.[13] Stories circulate of them arriving at births 'in a special carriage' and with 'a huge wooden box adorned with gilded carvings', in which their instruments were hidden.[14] A blindfold was placed over the eyes of women in labour and other members of the household were evacuated from the birth chamber when forceps were used. So long as the design of the new tools was concealed, it has been said, 'the skills of [the] Chamberlens, who carried out deliveries under a sheet or blanket, must have seemed almost magical.'[15] Substantial commercial interests buttressed these secretive practices. The prestige and financial benefits of having a monopoly over the use of this mystical tool were, at the time, considerable.

Although the use of forceps eventually extended beyond the Chamberlen family, the deployment of these tools continued to be restricted. As forceps were not considered the domain of midwives, highly gendered divisions of labour were operative and consolidated. The use of forceps is seen to have given doctors and surgeons a distinct advantage over midwives in the market for attending births, and by the end of the eighteenth century, they were supporting people through even straightforward births that would have previously been attended by midwives; they thereby emerged, for the first time it would seem, as *direct competitors* to midwives.[16] However, it seems unlikely that such a shift occurred purely because of the technologies these men wielded. Medical historian, Adrian Wilson, suggests that around that time, women of the upper classes – more literate than they had been previously and with considerable leisure time – were seeking to differentiate themselves from their exploited counterparts, and choice of birth attendant was one way to achieve that. In his own words, they 'abandoned the female midwife in an attempt to demarcate themselves from their humbler fellow-women'.[17] In so far as that is the case, the shift away from midwifery was not just about technology, but was intimately bound with class-based prejudice and ideology. Indeed, the tools themselves (particularly in unskilled or overly enthusiastic hands) were not as safe as they were revered, and they potentially facilitated the transmission and/or development of infection. This is suggested by the fact that from around the 1830s and possibly before, rates of death associated with childbirth were higher amongst the upper than the labouring classes, and even as late as 1930–32 this continued to be so; according to a prominent historian of maternal death, 'The only plausible explanation for this social class difference is that the upper classes were more often delivered by physicians and, therefore, more likely to suffer unnecessary interference.'[18] This was an era in which forceps were widely used by many doctors. The tools were not so magical for all, not even the middle or upper classes.

In 1920s North America, Joseph DeLee, who is now widely viewed a founding father of modern US obstetrics, contended that it would be advantageous for all women having a first baby, and many others, to undergo a forceps operation carried out by a skilful physician.[19] In legitimising the routinisation of forceps in straightforward labours, he argued that the labour of childbirth is inherently pathogenic and swore testimony to the gratifying results of his own approach. Although his approach involved a deep surgical incision of the pelvic floor (which was sutured with catgut after the operation), he contended that 'restoration of the parturient canal has always been perfect – indeed, nearly too perfect.'[20] DeLee was a prominent and powerful opposer of midwifery, arguing that the midwife is 'a relic of barbarism', and he added: 'In civilised countries the midwife is wrong, has always been wrong.'[21] At that time, many midwives in the US were Black women, Women of Colour and immigrants to the United States.[22] In the seventeenth century, midwives had been shipped from Africa to work as slaves in the southern states, where they attended the labours of other enslaved women as well as of the mistresses of plantations.[23] Following the abolition of slavery, many Black midwives had continued attending births in their local areas.

The subsequent erosion of midwifery in North America in the twentieth century was a profoundly racialised process, and it was far more extensive than in Europe. Given the celebration and promotion of forceps by those who vehemently attacked midwifery, the tools of the obstetric trade were deeply entrenched in highly racialised, as well as gendered or class-based divisions and relations.

This was not only the case for forceps. From 1830, surgeon François Marie Prevost conducted experimental caesarean operations largely on enslaved people.[24] Marion Simms, often described as the father of modern gynaecology, developed gynaecological procedures on enslaved women without pain relief.[25] He is well-known for inventing the technique used to repair vesicovaginal fistulas, a condition that can result from very difficult labours and that hinders a person's capacity to bear more children. As slavery and the production of enslaved peoples played such a pivotal role in the trajectory of capitalism, the obstetric and gynaecological technologies instilled in these women's bodies were inscriptions of the violent relations of a profoundly racialised mode of production. Unless that is emphasised, these people, their intolerable pain and enforced labours, are once again rendered invisible. Today, the names of these women, the few currently known from historical records, are beginning to be spoken and brought to the foreground of consideration. There was Anarcha, Lucy, Betsey .... In intensely political moves to reverse their erasure from historical narratives, they are now being acknowledged as the 'Mothers of Modern Gynecology'.[26]

In Aotearoa New Zealand, the dynamics through which obstetric technologies gained prevalence were intimately related to those which consolidated in the US and UK, whilst also involving trajectories of their own. The use of 'twilight sleep' in the first half of the twentieth century is illustrative in this respect. Twilight sleep was a powerful combination of drugs – often morphine and scopolamine – deemed to eradicate the pain of childbirth. In the United States, it was campaigned for by women (often relatively wealthy women) who were aware that it was being used in Germany.[27] Keen to be freed from the torment and agonies associated with childbirth, these campaigners protested against a medical profession seen as withholding liberation from them. In New Zealand, social reformers did campaign for its use on equity grounds, but the promotion of twilight sleep was also infused with ideologies of British imperialism in an era when fear was mounting that the Empire was in decline. The doctor who spearheaded the use of twilight sleep in New Zealand was opposed to the widespread use (what she called the 'abuse of') birth control in New Zealand, arguing that it had reduced the country 'to a dangerous state of stagnation' and, coupled with abortion, threatened 'to extinguish its white people'.[28] Twilight sleep, by contrast, was to be encouraged, as narcosis made it easier for British women to contribute 'to the nation's wealth' through bearing children painlessly: 'in the womb of British womanhood lies the Empire's progress and her strength', she argued.[29] As it turned out, twilight sleep did not entirely eradicate pain in labour, but it did erase *memories* of parturition, however excruciating the process and experience had been at the time.[30] Twilight sleep also had hard-hitting side-effects and hindered a range of physiological mechanisms integral to childbirth. Use of forceps became increasingly common as anaesthetised people were less able to push babies into the world. Infants were often born heavily sedated and struggled to take their first breath. An extensive range of equipment and technologies were required to monitor and manage the side-effects of powerful sedation. Increasingly, birth moved into hospitals where arrays of equipment were readily at hand.

If, as Evan Willis argues, medical dominance was secured as capitalism shifted from its competitive or laissez-faire manifestations to the era of monopoly, such a process happened in different ways in different parts of the world. In addition to state-instituted mechanisms in some countries (as discussed in the previous chapter), many other processes, elements and local determinations enhanced the significance and importance of the technologies that obstetricians deployed as they rose to positions of socially sanctioned authority. These included struggles for market shares, highly gendered and racialised divisions of labour, class-based prejudice and ideology, the violent oppression and exploitation of slaves, and the dynamics of imperialism, as capitalism reached across the world and countries vied for prominence within that globalised environment. However important the technologies were, they did not act on their own – they were used, produced, advocated, demanded and circulated by people who were deeply instilled in such relations and acted within those contexts. As birthing came to be congregated in large institutions – namely hospitals – obstetric tools continued to be infused with related dynamics, much as newly emergent elements also began to operate.

TECHNOLOGICAL FETISH

Scholars within the social sciences and humanities have reflected for decades upon the significance of obstetric technologies in late twentieth- and twenty-first-century hospitals. In the early 1980s, sociologist Barbara

Katz Rothman wrote of the 'medical model' prevailing in the US context, an approach which ideologically prioritises technology and people's bodies are themselves seen in that same light.[31] The body is viewed as a machine in need of technical maintenance and fixing, much like a car in a mechanical repair shop. Drawing partly upon Rothman's work, anthropologist Robbie Davis-Floyd wrote of 'the technological model of birth', which she later renamed the 'technocratic model of birth', as prevailing in US hospitals.[32] Davis-Floyd emphasises that the birth process is widely presupposed to be 'chaotic, uncontrollable, and therefore dangerous', and moves are made to establish control through the use of different tools and instruments.[33] Parturition is deconstructed, reformulated as comprising distinct component parts, each of which is navigated with a range of devices and pharmaceuticals. When such manoeuvres result in unwanted sequelae, more technology is used in efforts to improve on the situation.[34] Today the term 'cascade of interventions' is commonly used within clinical practice to describe a tendency for the use of technology to accumulate in labour: when the deployment of particular technologies produces detrimental effects, others are drawn upon to counteract or manage the effects of the first. Newly emergent side-effects are monitored, presided over and negotiated through the use of more devices, pharmaceuticals and apparatus. In short, there is a profoundly fetishistic faith placed in technologies: they are assumed to hold the solution to a vast array of problems, whatever complications they have created in the past, may generate in the future, or evidence that they are unhelpful.

I am not alone in invoking the word fetish to write about technologies in contemporary birthing care. Sociologist Louise Marie Roth writes similarly in her recent book:

> Technology fetishism … occurs when obstetricians and hospitals ritualize technological interventions and turn them into taken-for-granted routines. Then obstetricians, hospitals, and birthing women can see no alternative. Many contemporary parents can hardly imagine experiencing labor without an electronic fetal monitor beeping in the background and acting as the primary focus of attention in the labor and delivery suite.[35]

Marxist political-economist David Harvey describes fetishism as 'the habit humans have of endowing real or imagined object or entities with self-contained, mysterious, and even magical powers to move and shape the world in distinctive ways'.[36] The use of technologies to alter the world – or, for instance, change the course of a labour – is not in and of itself fetishism.

People have always used objects to change the world around them, and probably the flow of childbirth also. I find it hard to believe that women didn't make use of the world around them, in order to support them as they birthed. For Harvey, a fetish arises when 'we endow technologies–mere things–with powers they do not have.'[37] People might like to believe, for example, that particular objects have the capacity to ensure endless happiness or physical beauty. They might choose to assume that a particular device is able to resolve vastly social problems, without the root cause of the problems ever being addressed. For Marx, fetish occurs when the configuration of social relations which enables an object to appear as if with a power of its own, are rendered invisible.[38] As philosopher Slavoj Žižek summarises, 'in Marxism a fetish conceals the positive network of social relations.'[39]

Whilst Marx wrote about commodity fetishism, Harvey has written specifically on the fetish of technology.[40] He indicates that for Marx, when particular kinds of new machinery and technology are introduced into capitalist workplaces, productivity rises. That is to say, less labour power is required to produce the same quantity of commodities than was previously the case; or the same amount of labour power can be put to use generating more products than was previously possible. When an individual capitalist introduces such labour-saving technologies into their enterprises, they can sell the commodities produced at higher profit than other businesses are able to because the price of commodities is ascribed according to average levels of productivity and in the capitalist's own business, productivity is *above* average. In short, 'capitalists with superior technologies can expect to gain excess profits relative to the social average.'[41] They may come to the conclusion, Harvey indicates, that the new technology is the source of the extra profits they are individually reaping, and they would be to some extent correct. However, it would be wholly erroneous to assume that technology is the source of profit generally. For Marx, profit arises because workers produce more value whilst they are at work than the value of their wages, and so profit – to quote Harvey – emerges 'out of the social relation between capital and labor'.[42] Harvey goes so far as to argue that 'The idea that machines are a source of value is, therefore, the fetishistic extension of the very real effect of superior machinery in generating temporary excess profits.'[43]

Whatever the source of technological fetish, the competitive advantage that individual capitalists gain by introducing new labour-saving technology into the work place is only temporary. Competing capitalists are under pressure to adopt the same or similar equipment in order to boost productivity in their businesses also. As technological 'catch-up' occurs across one or more industries, the overall effect is for the value of commodities to decline (as value is determined by socially necessary labour-time), and the capitalist who first introduced the technologies into the labour process thereby loses their competitive advantage in the market. Capitalists are therefore highly motivated to seek, develop and acquire new technologies in their enterprises, enabling them to attain excess profits – at least for a while. The cycle is ongoing, and it is partly as an effect of such dynamics, Harvey emphasises, that capitalism is a mode of production in which technological change is rapid and ongoing. Certainly the nature of birthing technology has changed rapidly over the decades. Where emphasis was once upon forceps or twilight sleep, birth workers are today more focused on electronic foetal monitoring, induction of labour, caesarean section, etc. – although forceps continue to be used at times.

This point is returned to below, following consideration of a related aspect of Marx's work: his depiction of capital, and therefore technology within specific capitalist contexts, as vampire-like. Such a connective discussion is important, as it enables some differences, but also parallels, to be drawn between Marx's analysis of technology and labour in industrial capitalism, and the forms of technology which prevail within many contemporary birthing arenas.

CAPITAL SUCKS

In the early days of capitalism, the tools used by workers were *means of labour* in the literal sense of the term: they were the *means* through which workers achieved particular ends.[44] Marx was of the view that this changed as capitalism developed. By way of explanation, it is helpful to emphasise that workers can *produce*, as well as *use*, tools and technologies. Through what Marx called their *living labour* – their ongoing activity – workers make use of relevant tools, and in so doing are capable of bringing new products and new technologies into being. Marx described these end results as having already expended labour embedded within them – that is, living labour that has been turned into an object. He referred to the labour embodied in those products as 'objectified labour' – as 'dead labour' even. The relationship between living and dead labour can potentially be complementary and dynamic, as people work to make things that will support and help themselves and others, and perhaps wider species and the planet too. Marx saw, however, that under the control of capital, the relation between dead and living labour is predatory. Capital extracts more labour from workers than the value of the labour they receive in wages, and continually introduces new (labour-saving) technologies into the workplace which themselves accrue as capital. As the productivity of labour is increased through the introduction of new machinery across different arenas of industry, a number of dynamics thereby arise. Rather than means of labour remaining precisely that – the means through which labour achieves particular ends – the activity of workers comes to be 'determined and regulated on all sides by the movement of the machinery'.[45] Workers are reduced to connections between increasingly mechanised elements of a vast automaton. Perhaps even more pervasively, as the machinery contains the 'objectified' or 'dead' labour of the workers, but is used to further reduce the quantity of labour required to produce more capital, such technics are *a drain* upon living labour. Marx's understanding of capital as actively producing a reserve army of labour is relevant here, but so too is his understanding that within capitalism, wealth and capital accrue in the form of equipment, technologies and workplace infrastructure. In his own graphic words: 'Capital is dead labour which, vampire-like, lives only by sucking living labour and lives the more, the more labour it sucks.'[46] Machines and technologies assume and play a particular role within capitalism. In so far as they are produced primarily for the generation of capital, they become antagonistic to people and manifest as if with a power and life of their very own.

Marx was writing about the vast machines of industrial capital in the nineteenth century. He was analysing the labour of workers who sweated to produce and then service those looming edifices of machinery. He called those labourers productive workers in capitalistic terms, precisely because they *directly* generated surplus-value for capital, and their living labour was therefore overtly turned into capital. Marx wrote relatively little about the so-called 'service-sector' workers of the era, such as nurses, doctors, or teachers, although he did observe that teachers can be *productive* workers in capitalist terms, producing surplus-value too. That is the case, for instance, when a school is owned by a capitalist and, in addition to educating students, the teacher generates profit: when, to use Marx's own words, the teacher 'works himself into the ground to enrich the owner of the school'.[47] In such a commercial establishment, the fact that the owner 'has laid out his capital in a teaching factory, instead of a sausage factory, makes no difference to the relation'.[48] By this logic, birth-care workers employed in health facilities owned by capitalists are productive workers also – they directly produce surplus-value. They may not directly make pharmaceuticals or medical equipment, but they are intimately embroiled in vast networks of productive workers globally, many of whom do. To the extent that the healthcare technology generated by those wider workers is used in private business-sector hospitals to increase the productivity of the health workers there, it might be considered that such apparatus *is* capital too – dead labour – which draws from living labour in order to generate more capital (see below). Yet not all hospitals are private capitalist enterprises.

Some hospitals operate on a not-for-profit basis, and many are owned by charities, or are state-owned institutions. That is not to say that these organisations are immune to the relations, or impress, of capital. The technologies used in those institutions may not be capital in Marx's sense of the term, but the workplaces are very definitely, to draw upon the words of Marxist-feminist Susan Ferguson, 'inflected with the rhythms and paces of value production'.[49] Drives to increase labour productivity run through state-funded institutions as well as capitalist corporations. Efficiency measures are common within the voluntary and public sector, as well as apparatus to increase labour productivity. These service providers purchase pharmaceuticals and medical supplies produced in overtly capitalist (surplus-value producing) industries. Even not-for-profit organisations are increasingly expected to run at a profit. In the discussion which follows, I consider some of the ways in which the development and use of technologies within birthing spaces has been intimately bound with such dynamics. I begin by focusing on the techniques and practices of the 'active management of labour', which Irish obstetrician Kieran O'Driscoll introduced into birth care from around the 1960s.

THE ACTIVE MANAGEMENT OF LABOUR

O'Driscoll began developing the 'active management of labour' protocol when he was Master of the National Maternity Hospital in Dublin. In Ireland, the term 'Master' refers to a senior obstetrician who oversees the administrative and medical aspects of the hospital for a set duration of time: seven years. O'Driscoll's 'active management of labour' approach involved a range of technical products including pharmacological oxytocin, equipment for administering the oxytocin and a hook on the end of long handle (an amnihook) for rupturing the amniotic sac that sits around the baby. Used in combination with one another in specific ways, these technologies constituted the 'active management of labour'. His approach has been described as the 'zenith' of 'a pre-occupation with labour progress and length'.[50] O'Driscoll assured that when childbearing was managed in such ways 'every patient was delivered within twelve hours'.[51] In order to achieve this, the active management of labour was tightly prescribed. Maternity staff, and *not* the childbearing person, were to determine when labour had commenced. Once a professional diagnosis of labour had been made, O'Driscoll was of the view that the woman could be permitted to stay on the labour ward. Following that, the dilatation of her cervix (the neck of the womb which has to open for a baby to be born vaginally) was to be charted over time on a graph (often called a partogram or a partograph). In the words of O'Driscoll and colleagues, 'intervention was mandatory unless cervical dilatation exceeded one centimetre each hour'.[52] Such intervention involved amniotomy: a procedure in which the amnihook is inserted through the vagina to pierce the amniotic sac that surrounds the foetus. That was to be followed an hour later, in instances where the birthing person's cervix was not deemed to have dilated sufficiently, by the commencement of an intravenous infusion (drip) of oxytocin. This is a pharmaceutical version of the hormone with the same name (oxytocin), that enables the womb to contract and therefore labour to happen. The rate of oxytocin infusion was to be started at a specified level, and to be increased every 15 minutes until a maximum rate (and maximum amount) of the infusion had been reached. For O'Driscoll, each woman was to have 'a personal nurse' during labour.[53] If the birth of the baby was not 'imminent' after 12 hours of labour, a caesarean section would be carried out.[54] In that way, a maximum duration of labour was prescribed.

When O'Driscoll wrote about the active management of labour for medical journals, his protocols were criticised on various grounds. Concern was expressed that control of childbirth was being taken away from women in labour.[55] It was not clear that childbearing people wanted their labours managed in such ways, particularly if the trade-off for a possibly shorter labour was more painful contractions due to the use of pharmacological oxytocin.[56] The oxytocin hormone is produced in human bodies during sex and orgasm, and has been dubbed 'the hormone of love'[57] for the feelings of euphoria and attachment it generates. Intravenous pharmaceutical oxytocin has the effect of stimulating uterine contractions, but without the enjoyable sensual feelings. Synthetic oxytocin also has a range of side-effects which can impact upon both the baby and childbearing person, including overstimulation of the muscle of the uterus. Questions are also being raised regarding the possible long-term effects on infants of the routine use of pharmacological oxytocin in childbirth.[58]

The active management of labour has also been associated with the assembly-line production methods of Henry Ford.[59] Within Fordism, production is centralised, standardised and occurs on a mass scale, and similar can certainly be said of O'Driscoll's approach. The National Maternity Hospital was large: around 7,000 people gave birth there every year.[60] With his approach *in situ*, he considered there to be a relatively even distribution of births across different periods of the day, week and year. Aware that the 'delivery unit' of a hospital can act as a 'bottleneck' because it is a central location 'through which all mothers must pass', his highly standardised rapid turn-over methods (assuring all births within 12 hours of the onset of labour) assisted the hospital as a whole to 'be efficiently used'.[61]

Integral to O'Driscoll's own approach at the National Maternity Hospital were also hierarchical divisions of labour and strict delineation of tasks associated with the management techniques of Frederick Taylor.[62] For Taylor, work was to be efficiently distributed across organisations, with workers ascribed well-defined roles, supervised and overseen by management. Within O'Driscoll's operation, consultant obstetricians were to agree upon management policy for care within the institution.[63] The work of specific categories of doctor was clearly designated and levels of responsibility ascribed. There was a senior midwife – the Sister – on each shift, in charge of the efficient operating of the 'delivery unit'. A minimum of one midwife was present at each birth, and it was the job of student midwives (who were at that time registered nurses undertaking postgraduate work to become midwives) to provide 'continuous personal attention' to women through the duration of labour.[64] One student midwife was assigned to every room. At times, student doctors were also assigned the task of being with women through their labour. It is seldom explicitly stated, but the 'active management of labour' was the active management of two different forms of labour. It was the active management of the labour of hospital staff, as well as the active management of the labour of childbirth.

There is an argument that the active management of labour was essentially a management technique which imposed upon childbearing a production-like process. In the words of Barbara Bridgman Perkins, 'With primary goals of accelerating throughput and enhancing productivity in the labor and delivery unit, active management and induction were inherently managerial techniques that enhanced the development of birth as a production process.'[65] What I want to emphasise is that the active management of labour did not just reconcile birthing with *any* production or management process. Introduced were work structures and processes akin to those which prevailed in industrial *capitalist* workplaces. In developing this argument, it is useful to note that in his classic text *Labor and Monopoly Capitalism*, Harry Braverman emphasised that Taylorism imposed on production the specific priorities and unique perspective of the capitalist: behind the commonplace features of Taylorism 'there lies a theory which is nothing less than the explicit verbalization of the capitalist mode of production'.[66] An antagonistic relation between workers and management is presupposed from the very beginning. Workers are *not* in control of their own labour process. Their work is managed so as to maximise or optimise what can be 'obtained from a day's labour power'.[67] Taylor was not interested in workers producing just enough to pay the value of their wages: he expected far more than that. Tools and technologies were used to maximise productivity, and similar can also be said about the method developed by Henry Ford. Braverman also saw that Ford's assembly-line approach involved the replacement of 'craftsmanship' with a tedious 'repeated detail operation'.[68] Living labour was heavily determined by the machinations of the conveyor-belt. Due to the competitive advantage that Ford attained as an effect of his techniques, assembly-line production was in time effectively imposed upon the whole of the car manufacturing industry. Whatever the objections of workers, mass production became a defining feature of mid-twentieth-century capitalism.

The National Maternity Hospital where O'Driscoll developed the 'active management of labour' protocol, was not what one might typically consider to be a capitalist enterprise. It was a hospital originally founded upon charity donations, and when O'Driscoll became Master the hospital catered primarily for women who could not afford to pay for their own maternity care.[69] Yet once the active management of labour was implemented (maybe even before), the 'rhythms and paces of value production' certainly made their presence felt within the institution. Comparing data from the National Maternity Hospital with that of other hospitals, O'Driscoll calculated that the 'unit cost of production, relating salaries paid to nurses to number of babies born, was three times higher in other centres, although the level of remuneration was comparable.'[70] I'm not aware that O'Driscoll suggested increasing the wages of staff at the National Maternity Hospital because of their increased productivity. Moreover, the active management of labour appears to have spread to and across the UK, as pressure mounted over costs and budgets within the National Health Service (NHS).[71] By at least the end of the 1970s, neoliberal economic policy was advancing and the state increasingly oriented itself towards controlling spending in the publicly owned National Health Service. In the 1993 edition of his classic book *Active*

Management of Labour, Dr O'Driscoll contended that the efficiency of maternity units is 'of great practical importance in terms of public expenditure at current levels'.[72] Through the active management of labour, organisational methods akin to those most associated with the monopoly stage of capitalism, made their presence felt even within publicly funded birthing services.

Key features of O'Driscoll's approach continue to be used in obstetric units across the globe, but his method of active management is seldom followed to the letter. Institutions have often adopted the use of pharmacological oxytocin and the practice of amniotomy, whilst the one-to-one care in labour aspect of his protocol (which in Dublin was performed by the student midwives) is overlooked. In other words, reflecting the priorities of capitalist value production not least in an era of neoliberalism, it is precisely the use of the apparently time- and labour-saving technologies (such as pharmacological acceleration of labour) which have been prioritised; either as a deliberate strategy or due to workforce shortages, the provision of continuous midwifery support for a person in labour has effectively disappeared.[73] This is a significant omission, however, because research now indicates that continuous personal support is associated with a range of positive clinical and birth outcomes.[74] In addition to that, by the 1980s, O'Driscoll and his colleagues were of the view that their approach to labour management was responsible for lower rates of caesarean section at the Dublin hospital than was the case in many other – particularly US-based – facilities, but it was not immediately clear to which aspect of active management that was attributable.[75] When I first became aware of such questions, I initially assumed that if reduced caesarean levels were associated with the active management of labour, that would be a result of the use of pharmaceutical oxytocin and amniotomy. Perhaps this was not an entirely unreasonable assumption to make in an era in which technologies are attributed such high levels of import and power.

In a 1994 review of research studies on whether the active management of labour reduced rates of caesarean section and operative vaginal births (forceps and ventouse) for women having their first babies, it was concluded that active management does appear to reduce the frequency of caesarean births *but* 'the effective ingredient seems to be the presence of a companion in labour rather than the performance of amniotomy or administration of oxytocin.'[76] Two years later, after more research had been carried out, an author of the 1994 review contended that birthing units where active management was not practiced 'should provide continuous support in labour, but should not introduce the remainder of the package'.[77] The most recent systematic review of research on the active management of labour in relation to caesarean section reduction, notes that 'some components of the active management of labour package' may be 'more effective than others'.[78] To assume (as I initially did) that those components require tools or pharmaceuticals, rather than the *living labour* of one-to-one care, is to attribute more power to technology than it actually has.

I am not alone in associating pressures on staffing with the growing usage of equipment and technologies in the birthing unit. Thirty years ago, public health academic Sheryl Burt Ruzek observed that within maternity care, 'cutting-edge interventions involve the development and sale of machines – machines that are profitable to produce and market worldwide', whilst adding that such machines 'are marketed as a way to avoid labor costs'.[79] She went so far as to note that the 'entire medical-scientific literature is biased in the direction of assessing capital-intensive products over labor-intensive approaches' to birthing challenges.[80] A decade later, Barbara Bridgman Perkins indicated that within health environments, processes such as the 'substitution of capital for labour' have been supported by US health administration experts.[81] Through the ongoing years of neoliberalism, the substituting of technologies for labour appears to have continued apace. As the use of a vast range of obstetric technics has escalated, pressures on staffing appear to have worsened. A recent survey of midwives in the UK indicated that well over 80 per cent were unhappy with staffing levels, and over 65 per cent were unsatisfied with the quality of the care they felt able to provide.[82] The degree of industrial action on the part of nurses and midwives over the past decade is largely unprecedented and is attributable largely to inadequate staffing levels and burgeoning workloads, as well as below-inflation pay offers. Local communities are calling for change too. Pregnant people and families turn up to support midwives and nurses on picket lines and demonstrations. In the US, the Black Mamas Matter Alliance have called for 'providers and medical staff' to 'push back against a productivity model that does not give them enough time to build strong relationships with their patients'.[83]

CAESAREAN SECTIONS

Aspects of the 'active management of labour' continue to be used within many birthing spaces, but in capitalism, technological change is rapid and ongoing. Over recent years, it is rising rates of caesarean section, rather than the active management of labour, which has captured the imagination of many maternity service providers and commentators. The global caesarean section rate was 7 per cent in 1990; it is 21 per cent today and is anticipated to reach 29 per cent by 2030.[84] In the US, New Zealand and the UK, the caesarean section rate is – at the time of writing – above the 30 per cent mark. Today, the World Health Organization does not recommend specific caesarean rates at either national or hospital level, although the optimum figures that were widely cited within healthcare circles from the mid-1980s were 10–15 per cent.[85] Caesareans – 'belly births' as they are more fondly referred to – take place for many different reasons, including but not limited to the protection of physical health and the protection of a childbearing person's psychological and emotional well-being, not least after a previously traumatic childbearing experience and/or to avoid unsupportive 'care' in labour. Caesareans are *also* carried out for overtly economic and financial reasons which do not necessarily benefit the childbearing person or baby. In a document of World Health Organization recommendations, the Guideline Development Group noted that 'financial incentive remains a major determinant of caesarean births in all settings.'[86] In this section, I seek to identify and trace a range of political-economic and financial dynamics and relationships, which underpin the performance of many caesarean sections.

It probably goes without saying that many commodities are used each time a caesarean birth takes place: pharmaceuticals, infusion pumps, drip-stands, monitoring machines, antiseptics, surgical instruments, obstetric gel, suture materials, surgical masks and gloves, specialist lighting, surgical tables and more. When those products are purchased with a view to their utilisation, surplus-value produced by workers across the world is realised, contributing to the accumulation of capital in the hands of a few. Moreover, the pharmaceutical and medical tech industries have long been haunted by large corporate monopolies and quasi-monopolies serving to keep prices higher than they otherwise would be.[87] It is informative to consider these factors when reflecting on caesarean rates, but the points I want to emphasise extend well beyond that.

Left to 'its own devices', childbirth does not fit easily into a capitalist working day. In the words of midwife Denis Walsh: 'Just as it is impossible to pinpoint when labour will start, so it is impossible to predict its exact course or when it will end.'[88] It is partly for such reasons that O'Driscoll advocated the measures that he did, contending that his approach – not least in a large hospital – enabled 'peaks and valleys' in the flow of people through the hospital (associated with when their labours started) to be smoothed out.[89] As part of his schema, a core group of experienced midwives was assigned to staffing the labour ward at all times. Much has changed since O'Driscoll was writing, and as the safety of caesareans has improved, these operations are now a means by which some doctors are approaching the 'problems' of the uncertain timing of labour onset and duration. In the words of a private obstetrician working in Delhi: 'One normal delivery costs me at least a night, sometimes 2 nights. If I do 10–15 normal deliveries in a month I hardly ever sleep at home. If I do 15 caesareans I'm not home late for coffee.'[90] Particularly when doctors are working in solo rather than group practices (and so cannot call upon other doctors for back-up when work commitments collide), and perhaps especially when they need to maintain high caseloads in order to stay commercially viable, caesareans are a means of managing physician workload. In research conducted in the US context, there were higher caesarean rates amongst obstetricians working in solo, compared to group, practices.[91] Given this, it may well be that caesareans are a technology through which the labour productivity of obstetricians (in terms of births attended or babies born) is being raised – and if so, it appears quite likely that the income (and perhaps profits) of privately practicing obstetricians may be increased through the performance of pre-planned caesarean sections.

The World Health Organization is aware of the need for more research on related issues, and recommends potential movement towards staffing models in which care is provided largely by midwives with round-the-clock back-up availability of an obstetrician exclusively focused upon birth care.[92] One study in the US found that such a model reduced the caesarean section rate considerably, and was also associated with an increase in the number of people having a vaginal birth after having previously had a caesarean (this is called a VBAC: vaginal birth after caesarean). Aware that VBACs tend to be considered high-risk births requiring close monitoring, the authors suggest that such an increase might be due to doctors no longer having to 'contend with the difficulties of managing these high-risk patients remotely'.[93] Elsewhere it has been argued that 'many clinicians are unable to offer vaginal birth after cesarean delivery (VBAC) since they would have to be present throughout labor; under the laborist model, opportunities for VBACs increase.'[94] Yet it is unlikely that all doctors would want to work in such ways, particularly given the history of and ongoing animosity towards midwives in many parts of the world.

There is growing evidence to suggest that caesareans are more common within private hospitals than public hospitals, and that this is due to a range of reasons that do not necessarily relate to the choices of childbearing people. In the US, staffing levels appear to be a contributory factor. In a US-based study, people giving birth in for-profit hospitals were two times more likely to have a caesarean section than were those birthing in not-for-profit hospitals, after other influences – such as health and social factors – were controlled for.[95] The researchers hypothesised that caesareans were more likely to take place in for-profit institutions due to 'emphasis on short-term financial indicators, including payment of shareholder dividends'.[96] They anticipated that focus upon returns to shareholders would play out partly through the curbing of staffing costs, and indeed found that ratios of staff (especially full-time nurses) to hospital beds were lower in for-profit, compared to not-for-profit, hospitals. In discussing the relationship between higher caesarean rates and lower staffing rates in the for-profit sector, the authors suggest that birthing people may be more likely to engage in activities which physiologically encourage vaginal birth – such as walking, mobilising and changing position – when a nurse is present to support them to do so, than when a nurse is not available. I find myself wondering whether more caesarean births are scheduled in advance, enabling the (comparatively lower, and therefore cheaper) staffing levels to suffice. Yet whatever the mechanisms of immediate causality, there is certainly an argument to be made that births which take place *within* private-sector for-profit institutions are less protected from the 'vampire-like' tendencies of capital than are those which happen within the public sector. It may well be that the 'living labour' of health workers is more likely to be replaced by the 'objectified labour' embedded in the technologies required to perform a caesarean section, if a birth takes place within such an institution rather than a public hospital. In this respect, it is worth remembering that for Marx, in a private for-profit commercial business, technology assumes the form of capital, and capital draws from living labour in order to generate more of itself – in order that capital can grow.

If technology is used to increase worker productivity, and therefore profit, in birthing arenas, it is also pertinent to consider the role of finance capital in relation to such dynamics. Finance has been a crucial feature of the capitalist landscape since before Marx was writing, and he was acutely aware of its import in assisting the accumulation process.[97] Finance involves the funding of business and institutional activities. It often takes the form of credit loaned to businesses in order to facilitate continuation of their operations – such as purchasing and investing in raw materials, equipment and labour – when the company's own capital is caught up in other parts of the value circuit. For the financial sector, profit is made through mechanisms which include, but are far from limited to, the charging of interest on loans. Finance involves, to quote Costas Lapavitas, 'profiting without producing.'[98] Over the latter part of the twentieth century, the financial sphere of capitalism expanded well beyond the dimensions seen in Marx's lifetime, through a process often referred to as 'financialisation'. Marxist economist Paul Sweezy suggested that this came about in response to dwindling incentive, after the end of the post-war boom, for capitalists to invest surplus in mass industrial production of goods; they turned more, instead, towards investment in financial assets.[99] Whatever developments instigated the growth of the financial sector, within the US healthcare context, financialisation is closely associated with processes of corporatisation. Which is to say that, in the latter decades of the twentieth century, large corporations increased their ownership and control of key aspects of the health services (that might have previously consisted of smaller not-for-profit or privately owned enterprises) and developed substantial chains of hospitals and facilities. It has certainly been argued that corporate providers of the for-profit kind, encourage the provision of unnecessary medical services, tests and treatments, as investor profits are prioritised.[100] The authors of the article discussed in the above paragraph on caesarean rates in for-profit hospitals gesture towards a related point, contending that for-profit hospitals are quite likely to be part of a multi-hospital system, perhaps because they provide 'economies of scale'.[101] In that context, they add, care and staffing may well be standardised in ways that do not support the kinds of activities and staffing that actively facilitate vaginal birthing. Contemporary processes of financialisation also involve healthcare entities, be they of the public, private and/or corporate varieties, being transformed into 'salable and tradable assets'.[102] When hospitals are purchased and sold as assets, potentially between global investors, priorities very different from the well-being of childbearing people, local communities and health workers, are operating. The effects of such developments on various aspects of birthing, including caesarean section rates, merit closer research and analysis. There is now a powerful argument that the financial sector has become 'a structural determinant of health'.[103]

The insurance industry is also a component part of the financial sector that burgeoned into the twenty-first century, and caesarean section rates are known to be influenced by dynamics that relate to insurance. In many parts of the world, birth-care costs are paid for primarily through insurance and it is relatively common for health insurance policies to more favourably reimburse healthcare providers for performing a caesarean than for attending a vaginal birth. The World Health Organization currently acknowledges this, indicating that insurance policy reforms which more equitably cover the costs of both vaginal and caesarean birthing may well have a role to play in helping to reduce rates of medically unnecessary caesarean sections.[104] More than that, in various countries, private health insurers have tended to pay more for caesarean births than have public insurers (the latter being those which are directly linked to the state).[105] When insurance policies influence such details as whether or not a caesarean is performed, a largely invisible class of financial capitalists are involved (knowingly or not) with the intimacies of contemporary birthing.

Many birth workers are also dependent upon commercial insurance companies for professional indemnity or malpractice insurance. This is insurance which provides financial protection for health professionals (or their employers) if they are sued or if litigation is pursued on the grounds that they have made, or are deemed to have made, a clinical error. Depending on geographical area, such indemnity insurance is a legal requirement for specific categories of birth workers. In a study carried out in the US, high malpractice insurance premiums for obstetricians were associated with particularly high surgical birth and medical intervention rates.[106] The authors were of the view that these comparatively high levels reflected fear of litigation on the part of physicians in these areas. It has certainly been argued that, in so far as obstetrics is concerned, 'the course of least legal risk may involve surgical bias.'[107] Where insurance costs are particularly elevated, there may also be financial pressure on doctors to practice in the most cost-effective ways, and increasing c-section rates may be one way to achieve that. In the words of the authors of a 2013 report on liability insurance in the US:

> Available research suggests that cost shifting may be insulating net incomes of obstetrician-gynecologists from any increases in liability insurance and other costs. These analyses are consistent with recent trends in maternity care. Intensified use of childbirth technologies can generate revenue efficiently.[108]

It is also possible that insurers are placing restrictions upon the practice of birth workers which effectively prescribe the use of specific technologies. In the US, for example, it has been reported that some malpractice insurance policies do not include coverage for obstetricians who help a person to birth vaginally after they have previously had a caesarean section, with such an exclusion 'effectively forcing healthy women and newborns to undergo major surgery at increased cost to payers'.[109] The same report notes instances of additional insurance costs having being charged to physicians who work with midwives.

In other areas, a primary issue has been a generic lack of insurance for particular categories of birth workers. In the UK for instance, independent midwives (those who work outside of the NHS) have, at various points in time, struggled to attain professional indemnity insurance.[110] In 2014, it became a legal requirement for health professionals in the UK to hold professional indemnity insurance, yet adequate insurance has simply not always been available for the small number of self-employed midwives in the country. As one explained in 2021, insurance companies 'are really focused on profit margins. They need to be making money. At the moment, you know, a small number of midwives needing a policy isn't going to be providing them with a great deal of profit.'[111] The people who birth with independent midwives tend to have high rates of vaginal birth, so at times when these midwives cannot attend births there is likely to be upward pressure, however slight, upon caesarean rates. Home-birth midwives have faced related issues around insurance in Australia.[112]

Much has been written about obstetric technologies – including caesarean section – over the years, and often about their burgeoning usage which considerably outweighs need or even desire on the part of pregnant people. For Marx, fetishism occurs when an object, in place of the social relations which give rise to that object, are brought to the foreground of consideration. Through use of obstetric technologies, childbearing people and their loved ones are connected with workers in hospitals and factories across the world, with the capitalist owners of medical tech and pharmaceutical companies, with the owners and administrators of hospitals (which are increasingly managed according to capitalist-type principles even if they are public-sector institutions), with insurers, financiers and investors. I'm sure the list is longer still. Given the vast networks of vested interests, perhaps it is unsurprising that people often feel as if the technologies of childbirth have a power of their own: as if somebody else is pulling the strings regarding their usage.

UNCERTAINTY AND TECHNOLOGICAL FETISH

Within Marxism, fetishism occurs when the social relations which enable something to attain prominence are veiled, yet there is another reading of fetish which is also relevant to contemporary birthing. This is a reading drawn from the psychoanalytic tradition. Within such a formulation, fetish refers to an object which masks the impossibility upon which the symbolic order is premised.[113] Which is to say people may become preoccupied with particular *things* (objects of fetish) when they acknowledge, on some level, that their understanding of the world is imperfect and fallible, but simultaneously disavow that. By such an account, fetishes help people to feel safe. They are a way of holding at bay uncertainties which might otherwise make life feel overwhelming and to some extent untenable.

Childbirth is certainly an aspect of life that evades the certainties of the symbolic order. As a skilled and experienced midwife once shared with me: 'However many births you have been at, you have never been at the next birth.'[114] I have often reflected fondly on her turn of phrase and on her expression of impeccable logic which simultaneously oozes sensibility towards that which is neither entirely known nor calculable. She is not alone in gesturing towards the expansiveness of birth in relation to formalised knowledge. Some have used the term 'uncertainty' in signalling the tenuous but intractable interstices of comprehension and its absences. Canadian obstetrician Murray Enkin wrote of his sixty years associated with pregnancy care, culminating 'in a reluctant but comforting acceptance of uncertainty'.[115] Others have spoken about the 'grey areas' of intrapartum care in terms of that which is not entirely known, and in the words of a US physician, 'we're constantly managing uncertainty on the labor floor.'[116]

The birthing literature is replete with examples of technologies being deployed to guard against the incompleteness of knowledge. Anthropologist and physician Claire Wendland identifies a prevailing assumption within birthing spaces that 'technology magically wards off the unpredictability and danger of birth.'[117] Davis-Floyd indicated similarly when she argued that 'obstetricians and nurses who have experienced the agony or confusion of maternal or fetal death, or the miracle of a healthy birth when all indications were to the contrary' are aware, in some way, that complete knowledge and control of birth is beyond them.[118] By her understanding, technocratic rituals are the means by which such anomalies are resolved. The language of fetish resonates with aspects of Davis-Floyd's analysis whilst perhaps lending more credence to the deeply personal, as well as social or cultural, ways in which such repetitious attachments assume traction in birthing spaces. US obstetrician Neel Shah indicates the significance of this when he makes the following observation about a caesarean carried out to protect the unborn:

> ... if the baby comes out looking perfect and pink and squirming around, I think, hey, it's a good thing I did a C-section. I totally won. And if the baby comes out blue and lackluster, I think, man, it's a really good thing I did a C-section. So either way, it's pretty good to be me because I'm always

> right. That being said, you know, we think at least half of the C-sections that we do are probably not necessary.[119]

Whatever the outcome of the surgery it is understood to have been the right and necessary course of action. Yet there is nonetheless a lurking suspicion that such an outcome may *not* have been entirely essential. The impossibility of ontological certainty is configured in such a way as retroactively supports the performance of caesarean section *whatever the sequence of events that follows.* In this regard, the obstetrician's sense of who he is in the world is protected: 'it's pretty good to be me because I'm always right.'

Psychical protection of the self does not negate the role of political-economic pressures in shaping decision-making on the labour ward in a manner that suggests the role given to fetish. Shah is acutely aware that decisions over whether to perform a caesarean are made as clinicians manage the flow of 'patients' through hospitals. Maternity service workers may be caring for multiple pregnant people at a time, and trying to simultaneously ensure the availability of rooms and staff. In such conditions, a caesarean may well be carried out earlier than would otherwise be the case:

> So you can imagine that if you have three patients that you're caring for and you're totally out of beds on the labor floor. Every bed is full. And you really need to make a bed available. And one woman is taking much longer than average. And you believe in your heart that ultimately she's going to need a C-section anyway, you might do it an hour earlier than you absolutely have to. But the truth is in obstetrics, we never know. And there is many times where people eke it out.[120]

Once again, this particular caesarean section may not have been entirely necessary but it was carried out anyway. A c-section, Shah argues, is the frequently pulled 'ripcord' through which uncertainty on the part of practitioners can be exited.[121] He repeats: 'It's like your way out. It's your way out of the uncertainty.'[122] If technological fetishism involves simultaneous acknowledgement, and covering, of the impossibility haunting aspirations to achieve certainty in the arena of birth, it is a fetishism that is particularly at home in contemporary maternity units where there are staffing constraints, shortages of 'living labour' and pressures to increase the productivity of the workers who turn up on shift each day. But there is something that needs to be added to this discussion. And it is this: if one argues that technology *is* the problem which haunts contemporary birthing, there is also a danger of masking the dynamics of capitalism by which technology has achieved this standing, and of thereby fetishising the technological.

Pervasive combinations of desire and practice which support the burgeoning use of commodified technologies are more prevalent in some birthing units and circumstances than others. This is not to deny that they are widely normalised across many birthing spaces whatever their ownership structure and however the care in those places is funded. Such powerful preoccupations simultaneously affect how parturition is approached and birthing people are supported, as well as facilitating, being bolstered by and *masking* capital accumulation for medical-related companies and financial-sector businesses across the world. The dynamics are far-reaching and propelling, but despite the proliferating use of obstetric technologies, such equipment and technics are not available for everybody as and when needed. To suggest that this is the case because nurses, midwives, or birth workers are overly focused on natural birth, or are generally averse to using technology (neither accusations being particularly uncommon), may indicate once again that the social relations of capitalism are failing to be acknowledged.

TOO LITTLE, TOO LATE? OR CAPITALISM AS USUAL?

Even the Global North has 'maternity care deserts'.[123] Broadly speaking, these are parts of a country without obstetric facilities and they may also be without midwifery care as well. In the US, over 2.2 million women of childbearing age live in areas defined as maternity-care deserts, and 36 per cent of the US counties are described as such.[124] Many hospitals close and exit areas (thereby creating, or leaving an area closer to becoming, a maternity-care desert) for reasons relating to low or reduced levels of profitability. Such institutions are described as being 'financially distressed'.[125] Whilst dynamics pertaining to finance and profitability influence the *overuse* of obstetric technology, they also relate to many technologies not being available for pregnant people at all. In this regard, 'too little, too late' scenarios are intimately connected to those of 'too much, too soon'.[126] Perhaps neither are aberrations within the context of the current economic system, but indicative of capitalism operating as usual. A system which is driven by the accumulation of capital also creates vastly inequitable distributions of technologies and health services.

Childbearing people's access to epidural analgesia in labour has also been a site of contention, not least in the UK. In 2020, a series of articles were published in the media reporting on persons being denied epidurals when they were in labour. Article titles included: 'Women in labour are being denied epidurals by the NHS, amid concern over "cult of natural childbirth"' and '"I asked three times for an epidural": why are women being denied pain relief during childbirth?'[127] Factors which affect access to epidurals in labour are many and varied. Without knowing the details of a specific case in which epidural analgesia was not administered to a person who requested that, it is impossible to understand the precise dynamics which contributed to the situation. Having myself used epidural analgesia in labour, I am incredibly grateful that it was delivered swiftly when I asked. Yet widely operative presuppositions that responsibility for lack of access to epidurals lies universally with proponents of 'natural childbirth', are in danger of masking more than they reveal. Consultant anaesthetist David Bogod notes that staffing can be a considerable barrier to epidural access.[128] There will, of course, be times when the anaesthetist needed to put in an epidural will be in surgical theatre supporting a (perhaps emergency) caesarean birth, but Bogod is of the view that frequently shortages of midwives impede people from having epidurals. Given the potential side-effects of epidural analgesia, close monitoring is required and this tends to be carried out by midwives. Decades of neoliberal capitalism and austerity politics have resulted in a situation where there is now a vast shortage of midwives; in such conditions, many of the remaining midwives are concerned about the quality of care that they are able to give. One journalist reports on a woman's response to being asked whether she complained after not being administered an epidural in labour: '"Who could I complain to?" she said. "The country voted for a decade of austerity, so how can I be surprised by staff shortages?"'[129] If the monopoly stage of capitalism culminated in the provision of conveyor-belt care, in the age of neoliberalism it often appears that there are no longer sufficient workers to staff the conveyor-belt.

SYMPTOMS OF CAPITAL

The problem with birth care is not technology per se. As the subtitle of a key book by a widely published perinatologist suggests, there is a need for 'appropriate birth technology': that is, for helpful technologies, used and distributed in appropriate ways.[130] Marxism is not a tradition which romantically dwells upon the past nor encourages Luddite rejections of technology. There is more *gravitas*, contends American Marxist scholar Fredric Jameson, in beginning to imagine futures in which those aspects of today for which there is 'grateful and complicit enthusiasm' are preserved, at the same time as we begin to 'disintoxicate ourselves from the older system's powerful addictions'.[131] It seems to me that one prevalent contemporary addiction involves a sharp, gripping and incredibly alluring focus upon technology itself – an emphasis that blurs and thereby obscures from sight the many social and political-economic relations which give rise to the development and production of such technologies, to their inequitable distribution and usage. Tracing and highlighting such shifting, moving networks of interconnections is ongoing work. In 1994, it was noted that there is a lack of in-depth, documented, information regarding the precise networks and chains of influence which shape the availability and purchase of birthing technologies, within both private and public services.[132] I agree, and to some extent that continues to be the case. Far more detailed political-economic research on such dynamics would be useful, but I am under no illusion that the search for knowledge of that kind will ever result in complete and exhaustive understanding of the situation(s) at play. If the relevant relations are complex and changing now, as hospitals are increasingly purchased by the investor class, such dynamics and relations are likely to shift and change again. More than that, if childbirth to some extent escapes the promises of the symbolic order, so too do the networks and relations of capitalism. In the words of Jameson, 'every attempt to construct a model of capitalism … will be a mixture of success and failure: some features will be foregrounded, others neglected or even misrepresented.'[133] He notes that nobody 'has ever seen that totality, nor is capitalism ever visible as such, but only in its symptoms'.[134] This is another way of considering the TREC (technology-risk-evidence-choice) quartet: each element of the acronym appears as an obvious, a 'natural' even, starting point for investigation of childbirth precisely because it is symptomatic of the ways in which extensive networks of political-economic and social relations are currently playing out and consolidating. There are also operational linkages between the different elements of TREC. For instance, when the effects of particular technologies are unknown, formulations of *risk* have become a compelling and dominant way of narrating such uncertainty. A person may be informed of a one-in-a-hundred risk of a particular eventuality occurring as a result of the use of particular procedure and/or technology. But – and it's an important but – there are no guarantees that the person in question will or won't be the one in a hundred who experiences such complications. If it turns out that they are, they may be offered further technologies in attempts to remedy the side-effects generated by the use of the first – if, perhaps, they are lucky. Another risk ratio might even be presented to them by health professionals as a means of quantifying the murky waters of the future unknown. If fetish is a protection against the uncertainty which haunts human understandings and articulations of childbirth, formulations of risk are a means through which that uncertainty is powerfully and prevalently articulated. Perhaps calculations of risk also lend a semblance of certainty to circumstances which lack precisely that. They are another of the machinations of contemporary maternity units. Risk is the focus of the next chapter.

4
Subsumed by Risk

Much has been written about risk in pregnancy. A wide variety of foods and activities – from the eating of certain cheeses and the drinking of alcohol, to the changing of cat litter – are seen to pose risks for the developing foetus. If a pregnant person has a pre-existing medical condition or has previously had a caesarean birth, these are described as 'risk factors' for pregnancy-related complications. Within perinatal services, people are often categorised as being at high or low risk of particular outcomes. If complications develop during gestation, a pregnancy might shift from being considered 'low risk' to 'high risk'. There is a distinct absence of a 'no risk' category for classifying people with healthy pregnancies.[1] It seems hardly feasible to imagine childbirth today without some degree of risk. Birth, it has been said, is 'always and everywhere in our world understood as risky'.[2] The aim of this chapter is to begin to denaturalise contemporary constitutions of birth as risk, through exploring key relations and dynamics upon which such formulations depend. Risk is in this way demonstrated as a mechanism through which aspects of capitalism and of associated structures of oppression are able to operate without those broader contexts and relations being rendered visible.

In his now-classic book *Risk Society*, Ulrich Beck depicted the latter decades of the twentieth century as characterised by the rising prevalence of risk.[3] He saw early industrial development as having largely facilitated the meeting of physical human needs, but in time the benefits of technological and economic development came to be obscured by proliferating hazards and dangers, including threats of nuclear war and environmental collapse. Beck was of the view that science had traditionally focused upon perils emanating from 'nature' and the 'external' world, yet was now forced to face the dangers that science and industrialisation had themselves generated.[4] Whilst Beck acknowledged the need for restrictions on free trade in order to mitigate risks on a global scale,[5] he fell considerably short of questioning the basic premises upon which capitalism operates. If we understand many of the problems that Beck emphasises, such as the dangers of industrialisation or global financial melt-down, as integral to the very mechanisms of capitalism, risk can be formulated in very different terms.

In this chapter, I draw upon the Marxist notion of subsumption in order to make sense of the normalisation of childbirth as risk. Within Marxism, 'subsumption' is a process through which capital draws labour into its auspices, and in so doing transforms the very nature of work, of associated technologies, of the knowledge needed to operate and produce those mechanics, and of broader aspects of life upon which these impact.[6] As subsumption reached new heights in the era of late capitalism (broadly speaking from the mid-twentieth century onwards), various related mechanisms came to operate which progressively facilitated the saturating of childbirth by risk. Yet as capitalism is wrought with contradiction, so too I suggest are these processes. I begin by briefly locating the analysis of risk within historical context.

HISTORICISING RISK

Definitions of risk vary but broadly speaking, risk is the probability or chance that something will happen – usually something that is not desired. Risk pertains to situations of uncertainty, and designates the possibility of particular outcomes within those conditions. Modern calculations of risk are premised in the Hindu-Arabic numeral system which was introduced into Europe around the time of the twelfth century, although it was not until many centuries later that the study and analysis of risk really began to take off.[7] In the 1650s, a Frenchman with an inclination for gambling, Chevalier de Méré, called upon mathematician Blaise Pascal to solve a particular paradox relating to the chances of winning in gambling games. It is in this context that concepts crucial to probability theory, upon which contemporary calculations of risk are premised, were developed by Pascal and Pierre de Fermat (with whom Pascal corresponded on the matter). Around the time that a fledgling capitalism was beginning to take off, it therefore became increasingly possible to build and develop calculations of risk. American economist Peter Bernstein recounts such a series of events, arguing also that the 'capacity to manage risk, and with it the appetite to take risk and make forward-looking choices, are key elements of the energy that drives the [capitalist] economic system forward.'[8] He wrote these latter words specifically in relation to late twentieth-century capitalist developments, but I doubt Marx would have agreed with his argument. For Marx, it is the incessant drive for surplus-value on the backs of workers, rather than risk-taking on the part of capitalists, which serves as the motor force of capitalism. Marx wrote vociferously against the 'absurdity' of the 'bourgeois conception of profit as reward for risk'.[9] If goods produced by workers are not sold in the market place, those labourers are subjected to wholesale unemployment. It is workers rather than capitalists, he argued, who run 'the greatest risk'.[10]

This is not to deny that risk calculations were and continue to be extensively used within the institutions of capitalism. By Bernstein's account, they were widely deployed within a marine insurance industry that was burgeoning in London by the mid-eighteenth century.[11] By this point in history, he argues, wealth had ceased to be something primarily 'inherited from preceding generations: now it could be earned, discovered [*sic*], accumulated, invested – and protected from loss.'[12] I prefer to say that risk calculations became integral to the protection of capital and of wealth accrued by dispossession (through processes of so-called primitive accumulation) across the world, and were particularly important as the financial (including insurance) sector of capitalism developed.

It was not until much later that risk began to be calculated in relation to childbirth. Anthropological accounts emphasise a gradual shifting – at different times in different social and cultural environments – from birth being understood as to some extent beyond human control, to the recalcitrance associated with birth being scientifically formulated and configured as a site for technical manipulation: 'What was once the domain of chance, fate, or divine will has been repositioned as behavioral "risk," both scientifically calculable and technologically avoidable.'[13] Some scholars have suggested that focus upon risk implies a more 'activist stance' than previous formulations which emphasised birth as a 'dangerous event'.[14] I am keen to avoid presuppositions that historically people(s) across the world have not *acted* in relation to childbearing, and more specially have not acted in ways that enabled health and saved lives. To give just one example, recent historical work indicates that in England the outcomes of births attended by sixteenth-century midwives were far better than has previously been assumed, and may not have been repeated again before the twentieth century.[15] Nonetheless, there *is* an activism involved in risk analysis/management, and it is one focused upon the ascription of potential hazards and the performance of ongoing and continually pre-emptive strategies. Such a stance is particularly congruent with a broader context in which people are held primarily responsible for their fate, and there is a steady flow of means by which hazards can be identified and dealt with.

There are certainly references to risk in the birthing literature from at least the eighteenth century. In the 1760s, an eminent London midwife wrote of 'the risk' of particular eventualities when a breech delivery is 'ill managed'.[16] She also warned of 'the unnecessary tortures and risks' of the use of 'iron and steel instruments'.[17] Meanwhile, a prominent Scottish obstetrician wrote of instances in which women might not have 'run such a dangerous risk' were forceps used sooner.[18] Yet it was in the twentieth century that risk emerged as a pre-eminent mechanism for the active calculation of the possibility of particular pregnancy outcomes, and for the strategic differentiation of groups of women within a pregnant population. Since then, the pregnant population has apparently gotten riskier. In England, well over half of the birthing population (55 per cent) was recently calculated as being at 'higher risk' compared to 'lower risk' of complications (45 per cent).[19] Even in the Netherlands – a country well known for having a high home-birth rate in comparison to other countries of the Global North – the list of 'risk conditions' considered of relevance in deciding upon 'levels of care' (e.g., in a hospital or not), has grown substantially: the list contained 39 items in 1958 and 143 by 2003.[20] In the US, it is reported that 'life-threatening conditions that are chronic in nature and not directly caused by pregnancy, such as cardiac disease and mental health conditions, have been rising.'[21] Risk, it would seem, has piled upon risk, and 'complexity' (a commonly used word in today's maternity services) has accrued.

SUBSUMPTION

Perhaps it is not surprising that the word 'subsumed' has been used to depict the relationship of birth to risk. Whilst midwifery practice has long been regulated to focus upon 'normal' childbearing (as touched upon in Chapter 2), UK-based researchers have indicated that understandings of normality are difficult to sustain and 'easily subsumed by the linguistically and culturally more secure notion of risk'.[22] I would go so far as to say that birth generally has been subsumed by risk. In everyday terms, subsumption is a process through which something – in this instance pregnancy or childbirth – comes to be incorporated into a wider system or category. Subsumption has a more specific meaning within Marxism.

For Marx, the subsumption of labour under capital is a process integral to the very operations of capitalism. He differentiated between two categories of subsumption: 'formal' and 'real'. Formal subsumption is a process whereby capital takes over labour processes that were previously organised outside of capital, and thereby turns labour into capital.[23] Formal subsumption involves the appropriation of absolute surplus-value. That is the form of surplus-value sometimes associated with the early days of capitalist accumulation – although it is far from limited to that era – and it is produced when the working day is elongated beyond (and often well beyond) the time necessary for the workers to produce the value of their wages. In contrast, *real* subsumption occurs when capitalists reap what Marx referred to as 'relative surplus-value'.[24] This is surplus-value accrued when the length of time required to produce the value of workers' wages (or that required to ensure their livelihood) is reduced and so the proportion of time dedicated to creating surplus-value for capital is effectively increased.[25] This occurs through such processes as the introduction of technical developments in the workplace, and the transformation of means of production which boost worker productivity. *Real* subsumption requires ongoing technological changes across all sectors of industry, not least because if businesses are to remain competitive in the market, they must produce at similar paces and adopt related apparatus. Marx noted, for example, that the development of spinning machines (in place of person-powered spinning wheels) was inseparable from the development of power-looms which enabled fabric to be woven more quickly.[26] He posited changes in engineering as inseparable from vast transformations of shipbuilding. For Marx, real subsumption involves the continual application of science and technology – themselves products of labour – for the extraction of surplus-value.

Over recent decades, Marx's work on subsumption has been considered relevant to the various ways in which aspects of life, well beyond the arenas of paid work, are transformed in accordance with the influence and logic of capital. Within the autonomist Marxist tradition, Toni Negri speaks of 'the subsumption of the entire society under capital'.[27] As capital has expanded over time, subsumption is far more extensive than was previously the case and is ongoing in all areas of life. Federici, from the autonomist-feminist tradition, is of the view that from the end of the nineteenth century 'housework itself underwent a process of "real subsumption"'.[28] As the state's focus during that era moved towards 'increasing investment in the reproduction of labour power', work processes in households became 'for the first time' tightly bound with the demands and disciplines of capitalist workplaces.[29] In this chapter, I draw upon a slightly different reading of subsumption, and along with others I emphasise that the word 'subsumption' 'means rather more than just submission'.[30] Subsumption is a process whereby something is literally included or absorbed into something else, and in so far as this is the case, Marx's use of the word indicates that subsumption under capital occurs when something – labour – is actively transformed *into* capital.[31] In this respect, Endnotes emphasises that the 'labour process in both real and formal subsumption *is* the immediate production process of capital.'[32] Capital may be highly influential in people's everyday lives, however, 'Nothing external to the immediate production process actually *becomes* capital nor, strictly speaking, is subsumed under capital.'[33] I find this reading helpful as it allows for conceptual differentiation to be made between, on the one hand, the ways in which capital draws labour into itself (self-valorises) in order to grow, and on the other hand, shapes and makes its presence felt across many other aspects of people's lives. The deployment of labour power within productive labour processes – which can certainly include those of nurses and midwives employed by capitalists – directly produce capital and are subsumed under capital, whilst other labour processes or aspects of life are not. The latter, to draw on the terminology of Susan Ferguson again, instead reverberate with, and may indeed be submitted to, 'the rhythms and paces of value production'.[34] These might well be rhythms and paces very much in tempo with processes of real subsumption, but that is different from saying they have themselves been directly subsumed under – turned into – capital. In this chapter, I argue that childbirth has been subsumed by risk, *as* the real subsumption of labour under capital has continued apace, particularly in the latter half of the twentieth century.

KNOWLEDGE PRODUCTION: THE 'IMMATERIAL' MAKING OF RISK

By the mid-twentieth century, the real subsumption of labour under capital – involving the continual reaping of relative surplus-value and therefore ongoing technological change in factories, etc. – had facilitated a situation in which the production of goods was highly automated. Ernest Mandel observed that this was a period of capitalist accumulation in which machines were increasingly controlled by electronic apparatus.[35] Through the normalisation of Fordist assembly line methods in factories, goods could be produced on a mass scale, and over the decades that followed, such commodities as mass-produced washing machines, vacuum cleaners, televisions and later dishwashers became commonplace in many Western households. This was an era, following the Second World War, in which states in advanced capitalist countries also became more actively engaged in supporting the conditions which enabled the production and reproduction of labour power to staff the now technologically detailed production processes. In order to ensure productivity and profitability, argues Nancy Fraser, there was perceived need for 'a healthy, educated workforce with a stake in the system, as opposed to a ragged revolutionary rabble'.[36] She refers to this period as one of 'state-managed capitalism'.[37] State (and to some extent corporate) investment into aspects of life such as healthcare and pensions became relatively normalised, a development that the working class had been involved in pushing for.[38] Public funding of health research made much sense in this era, and also coincided with a movement within epidemiology towards the study of populations in order to identify factors operating at *the level of individuals* which potentially impacted upon their health (and which might therefore be modifiable at that level too).[39] The Framingham Heart Study is iconic in this respect. The US Public Health Service began funding this Massachusetts-based study and, whatever were the initial intentions around the study, it rapidly developed to trace a cohort of people over time in order to ascertain the factors operating in their lives which potentially contribute towards the development of cardiovascular disease.[40] From that research (which is still ongoing in much expanded form), it is now relatively common knowledge that smoking, and the presence of high blood pressure and blood cholesterol, increase the risk of a person developing cardiovascular disease; they are, to use a term very much associated with the Framingham research, substantial *risk factors* (potentially modifiable by individuals) for the disease.

This was also an era in which maternal mortality rates associated with childbirth had been improving and in the UK, concerns were being expressed that additional attention must be focused on reducing rates of stillbirth and of mortality amongst newly born infants.[41] In 1958, the British Perinatal Mortality Survey (supported by the National Birthday Trust Fund) was carried out, covering over 17,000 births in England, Wales and Scotland during a single week of the year.[42] The study identified higher rates of stillbirth and neonatal mortality amongst people who had previously given birth to a live premature baby, as well as amongst those who had previously had a stillbirth or a baby who died neonatally.[43] For women who had received no antenatal (pregnancy) care, the perinatal mortality ratio was five times that of the surveyed population as a whole.[44] There were higher rates of stillbirth and of neonatal mortality, and lower average birthweights, in cases where smoking had persisted after the fourth month of pregnancy.[45] Sociologist Lorna Weir notes that the initial report's authors tended to refer to the phenomena they correlated with perinatal mortality as 'factors', whilst also at times using the language of risk.[46] She contends, however, that by the end of the 1960s, the terminology had shifted and 'the host of "factors" that had been attached to the knowledge of perinatal mortality during the late 1950s and early 1960s … came to be named *risk* factors.'[47] As more research was conducted over the decades that followed, more information was developed regarding the types of phenomena linked to perinatal mortality and morbidity, and awareness grew of shifts in the relevance of particular factors over time and across regions.[48] This was also the era – premised upon those processes of real subsumption within industry – in which screens and computers came to predominate in many areas of life, at least in so-called advanced capitalist countries. Statistical techniques deployed by analysts were developing. Manipulation of vast datasets became easier – or at least more user-friendly – as, around the same time, deindustrialisation took its toll on sectors of the European working class and industrial manufacturing grew in parts of the world where labour power was cheaper. The late twentieth century witnessed a movement of workers in the Global North from jobs involving the production of 'things' into work focused on the production of information and data, as well as services. Terms such as 'information society' or 'information capitalism' came to prevail, indicative of the growth and prevalence of knowledge production around that time. Whether research was funded by governments, charities, or capitalist businesses, conditions were ripe for a veritable explosion of information on risks and risk factors: those relating to health and to various other aspects of life. It is within the context of such political-economic developments that much of the data pertaining to risks in pregnancy has been and continues to be produced.

Today, phenomena as diverse as emotional stress, a pre-existing medical condition, being pregnant with twins or triplets, eating particular foods, drinking alcohol, conceiving within months of a previous pregnancy, conceiving many years after a previous pregnancy, specific emotional states, being 'too young', being 'too old', being 'too thin', being 'too short', being 'too large', having a particular postal code, eating liquorice, and much more besides, have been gauged to increase risk (of one thing or another) within pregnancy. Some risk factors have a stronger association with unwanted pregnancy outcomes than do others and are therefore deemed riskier (smoking tends to be near the top of quite a lot of lists), and some studies are methodologically more robust than others. A phenomenon can be constituted as a risk factor for one outcome, but also an outcome in itself preceded by and associated with other risk factors. When specific factors are combined in a person's life, cumulative effects might be identified, indicating that the level of risk is raised above that attached to a singular risk factor. Of course, one course of action may be calculated as being more risky than another – and so it is relatively risky – whilst the absolute risk of that course of action may actually be quite low.[49] Some things are deemed to be relatively safe in one context or for a specific group of people, but are associated with raised risk in and for others. Perhaps it is not surprising that the list of risks in pregnancy often appears as if it were endless.

ACCUMULATIONS OF RISK: MONITORING RISK AND RISKY MONITORS

The production of information about pregnancy in terms of factor and risk analysis was always intended to have clinical applications. The authors of the first report on the 1958 British Perinatal Mortality Survey had advocated various measures across maternity care, including that anybody with a prior history of toxaemia (now known as pre-eclampsia), previous haemorrhaging in pregnancy, or caesarean section give birth in hospital under the care of a consultant.[50] In Weir's genealogy of perinatal mortality, she identifies the late 1960s as the era in which factor analysis was translated into 'a proactive screening technique focused on identifying the "high-risk mother" for the purpose of a more intensive regime of care'.[51] Screening procedures continue to be widely used within the maternity services as a means of facilitating identification of risk factors potentially influencing a person's pregnancy, and with a view to people being offered and/or taking up forms of intervention or procedures considered relevant in those circumstances. In addition to this, the proliferation of electronic goods in the second half of the twentieth century – facilitated by processes of real subsumption – involved the development and sale of new forms of medical equipment for hospitals. In the 1950s, metal or wooden horns (pinards) and stethoscopes were the primary means used by midwives or doctors to listen to a foetal heart during pregnancy. Over the decades that followed, a range of electronic foetal monitoring devices and machines became available and then widely used within obstetric units. The first electronic foetal monitor for commercial purchase appeared on the market in 1968.[52] In 1972, the NE4102 model of the ultrasound machine was launched, and it became the first ultrasound scanner purchased by many UK hospitals, as well as being sold in a range of other countries.[53] 'From the late 1970s onwards, ultrasound machines were medical white goods, standardised products in a high-volume global market.'[54] As electronic apparatus of this kind became commonplace within maternity units, it converged with the assessment and monitoring of risk.

Obstetric and gynaecological ultrasound scanning can be used as a diagnostic tool – as a means for identifying the specific nature of a problem, situation, or condition. It can be used to ascertain information including, but not limited to, the location of a placenta *in utero*, the number of babies in the uterus, the position in which a foetus is lying, and the presence of some conditions affecting foetal skeletal structure. Following the mass production and proliferation of ultrasound scanners, the technology began to be *routinely* used within gestational care – that is to say, when there was nothing to suggest any problems or heightened risk in a particular person's pregnancy. Operative therefore, was an assumption – which was not entirely new – that all pregnancies are, to some extent, risky. Today, ultrasound scanning is also used as a risk-assessment tool: as a means of ascertaining, in conjunction with information obtained from a blood test, whether a foetus is at 'increased risk' of having Down syndrome and other genetic conditions. The specifics of prenatal screening practices vary from one locality to another, but in a range of countries pregnant people are offered antenatal screening which involves the use of ultrasound to assess the thickness of the nuchal fold at the back of the neck of the foetus (a nuchal fold is often thicker if a baby has Down syndrome or one of a range of other genetic conditions), along with a maternal blood test.[55] Other factors will be taken into account, such as maternal age, and on the basis of that combined information, the pregnancy will be calculated as falling into a 'low risk' or 'increased risk' category. The cut-off between the two might be set at around 1 in 300 (policies vary: in some countries and/or areas it is higher and in others lower).[56] So, for instance, if the result of a pregnant person's test was calculated as 1 in 1,000, that person may be deemed to be at 'low risk' of having a baby with one of the genetic conditions being screened for, whereas if the result was 1 in 100 they are likely to be considered at 'increased risk' (the terminology of 'high risk' might be used). Given the assumptions of negativity that the word 'risk' carries, much could be said about disability rights and the framing of Down syndrome as risk. In some countries, it is encouraging to see that the results of these screening tests are being presented to pregnant people in terms of '*chance*' rather than '*risk*'. In the current context, however, the point I want to emphasise is that for pregnant people who receive a result of 'increased risk' or 'increased chance' as a result of the combined screening, the diagnostic testing offered – often amniocentesis – is itself known to generate risk: in this instance, risk of miscarriage. At the time of writing, the risk of miscarriage associated with amniocentesis was estimated on the UK National Health Service website as being 'up to 1 in 100' if the amniocentesis was carried out after 15 weeks gestation, and higher if it was done before that.[57] With the normalisation of ultrasound, as well as other forms of prenatal screening and testing, the number of sites at which risk could be seen to operate – perhaps unsurprisingly – grew. Even the development of Non-Invasive Prenatal Testing (NIPT), a newer, much more accurate, form of prenatal screening for Down syndrome – that is now available in many countries (although largely on a self-funded basis in Aotearoa New Zealand, at the time of writing) – does not entirely circumvent recourse to amniocentesis with the associated risk of miscarriage. This is because NIPT is not a diagnostic test, so there will still be a number of people who proceed to having an amniocentesis for diagnostic purposes.[58]

As the use of technologies such as ultrasound gathered momentum within pregnancy care services, the foetus was consolidated as a definitive, if controversial, site for the articulation of risk. That focus may be related, but not reducible, to the emphasis in the post-Second World War period upon protecting the health of the workforce into the future and upon reducing rates of perinatal mortality. Within this historical context, ultrasound machines facilitated visualisation of the foetus, and so obstetricians were able to cast their gaze beyond what Ian Donald referred to as 'the iron curtain of the maternal abdominal wall'.[59] With the emergence of the new technologies of the prenatal period, pregnancies that would have previously been viewed as entirely unproblematic could be aborted on grounds of 'foetal anomaly'. On the other hand, the foetus could also be studied and analysed in more detail than ever before. Physicians with a range of converging professional interests conversed over such issues as 'optimal' timing or modality of birth in different foetal circumstances, and the specialism of foetal medicine was born.[60] It is partly in this context that the foetus came to appear as if a 'patient' in its own right: one with not only risks and diagnoses, but treatments apparently unique to itself. With the use of obstetric ultrasound to guide them, doctors in time became able to perform surgery on the foetus in *utero*. As foetal surgery became a reality, a new arena of risk and risk management emerged. Surgery, and not least the foetal variety which *always* involves a pregnant person as well as foetus, is far from immune to unexpected and unwanted outcomes.

As ultrasound scanning has become a key tool in the formulation of obstetric risk, so too has electronic foetal monitoring. Continuous cardiotography (CTG) is a common form of electronic foetal monitoring, and the machines and devices that facilitate this procedure are a mainstay of most hospital birth units. CTG provides a reading of the foetal heart rate, as well as of the frequency and duration of contractions. Electronic continuous monitoring of the foetal heart is assumed to facilitate identification of circumstances in which a foetus does not have adequate oxygen supply and so needs to be born quickly, by caesarean for example. This form of monitoring is widely viewed as saving lives and mitigating risk, and in this respect is integral to the mechanisms by which risk is approached in contemporary obstetrics. Some birth workers certainly speak of being fearful of missing important information if a CTG monitor is not being used during a person's labour.[61] However, drawing upon reviews of existing research and a substantial retrospective study in the US, there appears to be a lack of compelling evidence of long-term perinatal benefit from continuous CTG monitoring in labour, in addition to clear evidence of high caesarean and instrumental (forceps/ventouse) birth rates when this form of intrapartum monitoring is used.[62] For some time now, various health professionals have considered the practice of listening intermittently to the baby's heart rate during labour to be as effective as CTG monitoring in so-called 'low-risk' pregnancies, and a recent comprehensive review of the research literature indicates a lack of robust evidence to support continuous CTG monitoring even when a labouring person has 'risk factors' operating in their pregnancy.[63] The authors conclude that 'High-quality research is urgently required to identify which women, if any, obtain a perinatal benefit from intrapartum CTG monitoring.'[64] What *is* apparent from the current literature is that continuous CTG monitoring in labour is associated with considerably higher rates of instrumental and surgical births (births by caesarean, forceps, or ventouse suction) than is intermittent auscultation (listening to the foetal heart at regular intervals). A caesarean, even in the absence of perinatal health benefits, may be unproblematic if the birthing person wants to birth by c-section. However, many people labour when, or even *because*, they would prefer to avoid a caesarean; surgery and instrumental births also generate health risks of their own.

Given the controversies which surround CTG monitoring, questions might be asked regarding why the practice continues to prevail, largely unquestioned, in many obstetric units. Causality is seldom linear, and there is no singular explanation which adequately accounts for current situation(s). Different types of CTG system are now available and used in different settings (e.g., in some hospitals, data on the foetal heart rate can only be read by people in the same room as the birthing person, while other systems transmit information to a centralised location on the ward) and such differences contribute to varying dynamics. Yet time pressures appear to be at play even if they are not determinant, across a range of environments. One midwife explained in the following way regarding her workplace: 'Sometimes you might opt to do continuous monitoring so that even if you don't have time to go near the mother … you can just have a look at the central monitoring and at least you will know that the baseline … is good.'[65]

Even in research carried out before centralised monitoring was implemented as widely as it is today, midwives spoke of using continuous cardiotocography in lieu of a midwife when staffing was short, and of monitors diverting their attention away from the labouring person.[66] Clinicians may gain reassurance from continuous cardiotocography, but it can also be a misguided sense of reassurance: more than information from cardiotocography is required to assess the well-being of a labouring person and foetus, and CTG traces can be interpreted in different ways by different clinicians.[67] In addition to this, if a baby is born in good condition via caesarean after a foetal heart-rate pattern has been identified as abnormal on CTG, people are understandably pleased that the baby is fine and credit may well be attributed to the CTG, not to mention the caesarean, as having protected the baby's health and life. It cannot be known whether the baby would have been born vaginally, an hour or so later, in good condition, if CTG monitoring had *not* been commenced.[68] In this context, perhaps there is little need to highlight that CTGs and associated instrumental births involve a range of products made in surplus-value producing conditions. The use of continuous cardiotocography on the grounds of risk management is just one of many ways in which risk and the mechanisms used to apparently control risk, are entwined – via complex arrays of interconnection, and even distant feedback loops and spillover effects – with the accumulation, not to mention rhythms and pulses, of capital.

UK researchers make a related point when they drew attention to the 'largely hidden, unacknowledged and unaccountable influence of markets … on our everyday construction of health risk'.[69] They contend that 'where health is framed by a constant expectation of danger, there is money to be made in providing investigative, preventative or curative products to counteract the risks.'[70] Perhaps in more Marxist terms, the contemporary prevalence of risk within contemporary maternity care is simultaneously facilitated by, and facilitative of, the accumulation of capital across the world. Yet that is not to suggest that technologies such as CTG would necessarily be superfluous in a non-capitalist society. Much would depend upon the specific dynamics and relations of the social formations involved. Perhaps, however, in a political-economic system where social good was prioritised over profit, the creation of more effective technologies than CTG might be prioritised.

As capitalism expands so too does capitalism's scope to actively generate health problems, whilst simultaneously producing 'responses' (effective or not) to those challenges. For instance, a range of pathologies are now far more common amongst childbearing people than they have historically been. This is partly due to the shifting contours and precarious nature of many people's living conditions in contemporary capitalism, while also influential is the production of new tools and stipulations of diagnosis. The age of childbearing has risen too, in some degree as an effect of economic constraints as wages have been suppressed through the decades of neoliberalism, and also because a widening range of contraceptive products – not to mention fertility treatments – have been developed and released for sale in the market. So-called 'advanced maternal age' is now categorised as a 'risk' for pregnancy complications – a risk factor associated with a growing section of the childbearing population.

INSURING AGAINST RISK?

Industrial labour has long been subsumed under capital, but as that process continued apace through the twentieth century and capital increasingly sought to make money from non-productive sources as well, the insurance industry was – as discussed in the previous chapter – integral to the rapidly growing financial sector. By 1989, there were well over 2,000 life insurance companies operating in the US alone.[71] Insurance companies are also integral to the proliferation of risk-related concerns within maternity care services. The fact that many health workers are today required to purchase and/or be covered (e.g., through their employer) by insurance of the professional indemnity or malpractice variety, has considerable significance in capitalism, because responsibility for the costs of raising children is structurally located with individuals and household units rather than with capital. As employers keep wages as low as is socially feasible, the costs of caring for a child who has been injured in specific ways at birth can be incredibly difficult for working-class families to afford. For instance, some babies are born with cerebral palsy, and in a minority of cases, the condition is the effect of actions or inactions on the part of birth workers. In 2003 it was calculated that for a baby born with cerebral palsy in the United States, the lifetime costs directly associated with the condition – over and above other living costs – were nearly $1 million.[72] Such costs will have risen since. Litigation against a health provider may be the primary means of families securing the money to care for a baby with serious birth injuries as they grow into adulthood, particularly in countries where no-fault compensation schemes do not operate. Disability rights activists have long argued that a person may be born with physical impairments, yet *disability* pertains to the *social arrangements and prejudices* which constrain that person's access to activities and limit their participation in life.[73] The fact that in contemporary capitalism it may be only if fault can be proved on the part of birth workers (or health system failures) that a legal case can be won and substantial economic support thereby made available for people with impairments, illustrates the intensely *disabling* character of contemporary capitalism. If blame *is* located with a health worker in a litigation case, an insurance company may cover costs that would otherwise be difficult (or even impossible) for the healthcare provider to afford. Insurance can therefore reduce financial risk for health workers or their employers, and to some extent for families, but that is not the same as making birth safer or ensuring that people's needs are met. Such dynamics are not entirely circumvented in regions and localities where no-fault compensation schemes are in place. It has been noted, for example, that even though a 'no-fault' compensation scheme is operative across Aotearoa New Zealand, the process of making a successful claim pertaining to infant birth injury can still require considerable searches for causality and may well involve identification of clinician error.[74]

Insurance practices create a range of challenges in relation to birth care. In the US, not only do instances exist in which insurance policies have been found to exclude cover, or to involve surcharges, for practices based upon solid research evidence, such as the provision of clinical support for vaginal birthing after somebody has previously had a caesarean section.[75] The very existence of professional negligence insurance has also been linked with the pursuit of litigation. It has been argued, for instance, that in the US when 'physicians sought liability insurance', they not only 'mitigated their individual risk' but also rendered 'each and every insured medical professional a financially worthy prospect for medical litigation'.[76] Most law firms are also businesses, meaning there is financial incentive for them to pursue clinical negligence cases, especially if such cases are likely to be won. There is now considerable literature indicating that fear of litigation on the part of paid birth workers is contributing towards 'defensive practice' – that is, towards clinicians acting 'to avoid liability rather than to benefit the patient'.[77] Concern has been expressed that once health service workers have spent considerable time placing 'ticks in all of the risk boxes' in order to fulfil hospital insurance obligations, as well as 'government targets', it is not difficult for them to lose sight of the person who is giving birth.[78] In the words of a UK midwife, 'risk management is actually stopping us caring.'[79] In short, risk assessment within birthing settings can readily merge into risk-management practices of a financially related variety. In so far as risk in childbirth is concerned, the profit margins of insurance companies – and to some extent law firms – are not to be forgotten.

The dynamics which fuel defensive practice extend well beyond those pertaining to insurance-related risk calculations and medical litigation. Wider interactions such as employment relations and state-associated regulatory mechanisms, also come into play. Depending upon the part of the world in which midwives are working, their actions are quite likely to be governed by a regulatory body established through state mechanisms. Investigations into clinical practice on the part of such an authority can involve loss of income for the practitioner under review and are often distressing, even though a conclusion may be reached that the clinician was not at fault. Such mechanisms apparently designed to protect public safety and ensure accountability can readily morph into channels of incrimination. In England, a veritable culture of blame or fear is seen to pervade both the perinatal services and the nursing and midwifery regulatory authority itself.[80] The term 'witch-hunt' is also used across a range of countries to describe investigations into the work of midwives (and sometimes obstetricians) who may well practice very safely but *do not ground their work in prevailing obstetric norms*.[81] Federici's analysis of witch-hunts as a constitutive feature of capitalism has been drawn upon to contextualise investigations of this kind, suggesting that such processes be viewed as examples of ongoing structural violence against women who challenge prevailing reproductive practices and norms.[82] It is partly due to punitive pressures operating within birthing services that various midwives claim to practice defensively; in ways aimed at protecting themselves from such interrogations and sanction.[83] Defensive practice can take different forms and may well involve clinicians deploying more medical tests and interventions than would generally be considered necessary for the well-being of the pregnant person – 'just in case'. Operative is an exaggerated attempt to avoid 'missing something' (e.g., a clinical detail) or to circumvent any developments that might have negative repercussions on the clinician. As a New Zealand-based midwife explained: 'you would practice defensively, you would send them [a pregnant person] for a blood test, or you would do a CTG, at every point where you think oh I'd better do that, better get the scans, I just need to cover myself.'[84] There is common-sense logic to such actions within social and historical contexts permeated by assumptions that medical technologies invariably mitigate risk. Yet it is not possible to plan for every eventuality in pregnancy and birth, and defensive practice is not the same as safe practice. Defensive practice generates a range of problems – risks even – including iatrogenic effects of overtreatment and failure on the part of practitioners to admit when they *have* made a mistake.

RISKY CONTRADICTIONS

If birth workers find themselves fearfully occupying environments subsumed by risk, they are far from alone in that respect. Much has been written on how pregnant people experience fear and anxiety as an effect of the dynamics of risk within perinatal services.[85] Individual pregnant people are frequently held – and hold themselves – responsible for the health and outcomes of their pregnancies. Yet risk involves numbers, or even generalised ideologies, indicating possibilities that may never happen. Being informed that there is a 1-in-250 risk of a particular eventuality happening during pregnancy, does not in and of itself enable a decision about an appropriate course of action to be made. Philosopher Slavoj Žižek argues that within so-called 'risk society', people continually find themselves having to make decisions that will crucially impact their lives, whilst simultaneously being without what he calls 'a proper foundation in knowledge'.[86] Thereby generated, he contends, are forms of 'radical openness and uncertainty' that can be intensely anxiety provoking.[87] Within birthing spaces, it is entirely possible for a person to 'have' a particular risk factor during pregnancy and yet never develop the associated undesirable outcome. It is also possible for a person to not 'have' that risk factor but to nonetheless proceed to develop said complication. The decisions that people make within birth care are seldom, if ever, premised upon knowledge of precisely what will happen as the result of a particular course of action. More than that, sociologist Jo Murphy-Lawless indicates that while risk has been increasingly used to define different aspects of pregnancy – 'in a mistaken attempt to cover all possibilities' – a situation has arisen in which the childbearing body has become more and more 'risk-laden' and therefore 'the possibilities for something "going wrong" proliferate.'[88] One might add to Murphy-Lawless' analysis that the more sites at which risk is calculated and at which possibilities for something to 'go wrong' are ascribed, the more sites are generated at which 'radical openness' and potential anxiety might also operate.

Most would consider some degree of apprehension to be normal in pregnancy, and there are many social dynamics (some of which sit well beyond pregnancy service contexts) that contribute to perinatal anxiety. Yet the contemporary prevalence of risk formulations does not entirely alleviate the pressures, and may even exacerbate them. Midwives are certainly very aware of anxiety amongst the people they care for, and in research carried out in Aotearoa New Zealand, they emphasised the need for extra support around this for pregnant people they work with. One midwife mentioned receiving text messages such as "'I did this and it made me worried" and "Did I hurt the baby[?]" and "Do you think if I did this and did that, and ate this and it wasn't hot enough then … ?'"[89] Some birth workers grapple with whether it is helpful to respond to such anxieties on the part of pregnant people by offering additional screening tests. Test results can themselves be unsettling, not least as they too are often inconclusive. As risk analysis has expanded through the pregnancy services, prenatal anxiety and psychological stress are now explored as risks in their own right. They are thought to be operative, for example, in the network of factors which contribute to premature birth or low birthweight in babies.[90] If risk generates anxiety and anxiety itself is deemed risky, it seems appropriate that questions are now being posed regarding *the risks of risk itself* and on the 'nocebo' (harmful) effects of risk labelling.[91]

In Aotearoa New Zealand, Māori scholars have written in extension of this point, emphasising the 'high price of being labelled high-risk'.[92] They indicate that formulations of Māori as both 'at risk' and 'high risk' coalesce with a range of prevailing colonial and racist assumptions regarding responsibility, vulnerability and capacities for change.[93] When these risk categorisations are used to describe and classify individuals in service-provision contexts, a range of social prejudices are thereby reiterated; and the very process of such risk labelling may even have the effect of actively deterring or impeding Māori from health service engagement. The researchers advocate a 'shift [of] attention from the individual to the distal socio-economic determinants which create lack of housing, education, employment – and the social system which fails to provide these things for Māori people to the same level that non-Māori enjoy'.[94] They call for a move away from formulations of risk that individualise responsibility for situations of inequity. Advocated instead is movement towards, and advocacy of, approaches capable of effectively challenging the social, cultural and political-economic contexts within which risk prevails and is unevenly distributed. Much work is now ongoing in Aotearoa which actively centres pregnancy and whānau wellness through

Māori ways of being and knowing.[95] This is very different from formulations of health which focus upon risk.

The contradictory and coercive dimensions of risk labelling are beginning to be taken seriously by some health- and birth-care workers. There is awareness that not all people perceive risks in the same way, and that something viewed as a risk by one person or social group may not be seen as risky, or be risky, for another. There is some understanding that risk can be used as 'a scare tactic' to coerce people into accepting particular institutional processes, procedures, or interventions.[96] Yet in various countries, increasing numbers of people are deliberately birthing at home *without* medical or midwifery attendance, and in some cases this is to avoid the effects of risk logics as they prevail within maternity-service contexts. In an article reporting on the experiences of women who decided to birth without a midwife or health professional in attendance, the researchers explain that:

> Fearful behaviours of practitioners for themselves created a situation where participants felt that midwives and institutional safety was prioritised over their personal circumstances, and that their beliefs, plans, and preferences for birth were subsumed by the institutional mood of fear. The notion of risk served to fuel this atmosphere … .[97]

The management of risk in childbirth is widely considered to make birthing safer, but it can also be a mechanism through which the oppression of women and childbearing people continues within conveyor-belt approaches to perinatal care which protect the medical institution. In this way, some people are actively pushed away from using the 'maternity' services. Perhaps it is unsurprising that such a situation was exacerbated during the COVID-19 pandemic, when hospitals were widely understood as 'risky places to be avoided', and increased numbers of pregnant people considered birthing at home unattended by health professionals.[98]

'PRISONERS OF THE PROXIMATE'[99]

Talk at the level of risk and risk factors renders invisible powerful social relations and dynamics. Sociologist Lorna Weir observes that when '[r]isk factor epidemiology' emerged in the latter half of the twentieth century, it 'formed a particulate plane of tiny concepts, a surface that displaced the depth explanations of social medicine'.[100] Risk factors are 'a measure of association rather than a cause', and they are constituted as operating primarily at the level of the individual.[101] In short, consideration of risk factors does not necessitate analysis of social formations and social structures, however influential those are in determining health. Importantly, one of the key figures historically associated with the development of *social* understandings of medicine is Engels. In *The Condition of the Working Class in England*, Engels attributed a range of diseases to the living conditions that the working class endured which, as Marxist sociologist Waitzkin notes, included 'malnutrition, inadequate housing, contaminated water supplies, and overcrowding'.[102] Engels traced various manifestations of childbearing or infant ill-health to the environments within which working-class women and girls were labouring and living. His approach was very different from the focus upon risk factors which prevails today. It was premised upon an understanding of capitalism as a vast and burgeoning totality generative of such conditions.

If all childbearing is today subsumed by risk, the working class continue to be disproportionately subject to childbearing complications and mortality. Preterm birth and stillbirth are associated with poverty.[103] To use terminology which prevails in contemporary epidemiology, people who are socio-economically disadvantaged are at higher risk of various pregnancy and birth complications – including serious maternal morbidities – than are other social groups.[104] Capitalism is also highly racialised and even controlling for indicators of social class, white women are privileged when it comes to mortality rates associated with pregnancy. If the role of intensely social structures in determining well-being and ill health is to be taken seriously, analysis *must* extend well beyond consideration of individual risk factors. More expansive analysis is needed to challenge approaches to birth and health which keep us, in various ways, 'prisoners of the proximate'.[105]

The approach to the analysis of risk I have developed in this chapter rests upon the premise that the contemporary constitution of childbirth in terms of risk is inseparable from the apparently 'distal' processes of labour's subsumption under capital. Without land, workers across the world have laboured to produce unprecedented volumes of commodities, technologies and resources which have accumulated as capital, and as they did so, the social conditions and technical composition of society were substantially changed. A range of possibilities emerged and/or expanded. These included new technologies, the potential for capital to make profit from non-industrial sources, and forms of knowledge production and data analysis that had not previously been possible. Such processes were crucial to the subsumption of childbirth by risk. Information, machines and devices for measuring and management of risk proliferated. Vast socially produced inequities came to be defined in terms of individualised risk factors and it might even be said that risk in pregnancy became a 'proximate' measure for the interests of a corporate and increasingly financial elite. Yet however 'risky' situations in childbirth are understood to be, that is not the same as knowing the best course of action to take in particular circumstances. The form of research deemed optimal for establishing the most effective forms of clinical practice, is the focus of the next chapter.

5
The Gold Standard of Evidence

Obstetrics does not have a strong historical record of producing scientific evidence which proves the health benefits of its own procedures and technologies. As surgeons and doctors sought to rival long-standing birthing practices such as midwifery, their claims to superiority were in no way *proven.* Before the early decades of the twentieth century, the use of forceps may have symbolised scientific progress whilst frequently ushering in more harm than good. At the end of the 1970s in London, Dr Archie Cochrane criticised his obstetric and gynaecological colleagues for introducing a plethora of procedures and processes into pregnancy and birth care without thorough evaluation of their effects.[1] He said they had failed to scientifically establish whether it was wise for pregnant women deemed low-risk to universally birth in hospitals. He spoke in complimentary terms about the British Perinatal Mortality Surveys and praised obstetricians for their involvement with inquiries into maternal mortality, but was concerned that these doctors had welcomed such developments as ultrasound, foetal monitoring and induction of labour without proper evaluation of the strengths and weakness of these tools. Since Cochrane criticised his obstetric and gynaecological colleagues over forty years ago, many women, parents, midwives, nurses, doctors, birth activists, etc., have rallied behind calls for what is widely referred to as evidence-based care or evidence-based medicine. In the words of a contemporary medical anthropologist:

> Evidence-based medicine is an important, if belated, contributor to clinical practice. The premise, that medical interventions should be proven effective before use, should have been key to obstetrics many years ago and could perhaps have prevented such missteps as the adoption of electronic fetal monitoring.[2]

Whilst many practices persist within birth care in the absence of clear evidence regarding their benefits, it would not be popular either amongst health professionals or birth activists to explicitly position oneself as anti-evidence. In this respect, evidence has become highly normalised within birth-care contexts: 'naturalized as self-evident and ahistorical'.[3]

When Cochrane called for his obstetric and gynaecological colleagues to develop and use evidence, it was specifically Randomised Controlled Trials that he had in mind. In their simplest form, RCTs are experiments in which research participants are randomly allocated to two groups and members of one group are given a specific treatment or intervention whilst those in the other group are not. Those in the second group receive a different treatment/intervention, which might be that which is routine practice in medicine at the time or a placebo. The latter set of people constitutes the control group of the study and the treatment being trialled is evaluated through comparison of measured outcomes between the two groups. RCTs are a form of research design well suited to evaluating pharmaceuticals. As UK midwife Sara Wickham has noted, 'if we discover a new drug which we think will treat a certain pathological condition, there is no better test of this at the current time than to conduct a randomised controlled trial'.[4] RCTs are important, and not least in an era in which pharmaceutical companies are powerful players in global markets. A 1948 study of streptomycin to treat pulmonary tuberculosis is widely considered to have been the first Randomised Controlled Trial within medicine – or at least the first that was reported on. RCTs developed a reputation for being a reliable means of testing a range of medical treatments and interventions, and in the 1980s the term 'gold standard' started to be used in the medical literature to describe RCTs in comparison to other forms of research.[5] This became a somewhat ubiquitous descriptor of RCTs, to the extent – it has been said – that they were constituted as 'a self-evident starting point in diagnostic or therapeutic evaluation'.[6] When a particular phenomenon is considered self-evident, that is often a clue that it has been significantly naturalised and normalised: constituted, in Marx's terms, as a 'concrete' feature of an intensely social landscape.

In this chapter, I consider a range of dynamics and relationships which supported the evidence-based medicine movement to emerge at the point in history that it did, and within that context for such prestige to be attributed to the RCT. I then discuss a number of limitations to knowledge produced via RCTs, and in so doing I focus in particular upon a specific RCT that has been well-discussed within the birthing literature: the oft-dubbed 'Term Breech Trial'.[7] The purpose of this chapter is not to denounce RCTs as an inherently 'bad thing', but rather to point to some of the ways in which their reified status in the production of authoritative knowledge has been intimately bound with capitalist developments.

CONTRIBUTORY FACTORS AND DYNAMICS

Historically, doctors have assumed considerable control over their own working practices and, from at least the early twentieth century, over those of other health occupations as well. By the latter decades of the twentieth century, some of that authority appeared to be waning. Whereas many doctors had historically been self-employed or owners of their own healthcare facilities, significant numbers were now earning a salary, employed in large institutions or corporations. Whilst some argued that medicine had been proletarianised, Marxist sociologist of medicine Vicente Navarro disagreed.[8] Medicine, he contended, has a controlling function within capitalist society which the proletariat simply does not have; doctors have frequently failed to support working-class struggles to transform medicine and whilst there are progressive and socialist physicians, what is happening within the profession is inaccurately depicted as proletarianisation. Nonetheless, he agreed that the medical profession was losing power and autonomy. Proletarianisation or not, calls for doctors to justify their clinical practice through using and developing evidence, certainly indicated that their authoritative decision-making capacity was not to be considered infallible or absolute.

Neither was that of pharmaceutical companies. The discovery of antibacterial sulphonamides in the mid-1930s marked an important development in relation to the reduction of maternal deaths associated with childbirth. It is also widely viewed as the beginning of the 'golden age' of drug development.[9] An outpouring of new drug discoveries flowed over the years that followed, and the pharmaceutical industry boomed. Not coincidentally, this period largely corresponded, and certainly overlapped substantially, with that which Mandel dubbed the beginnings of late capitalism, in which he argued that electronic machines became increasingly predominant across different areas of political-economic activity. Such technological developments are certainly acknowledged as facilitating the growth of the pharmaceutical industry during this time: its 'golden era' is said to have been supported by electronic instrumentation and 'underpinned by improvements in computers and their growing use in industry'.[10] The period of rapid drug innovation is broadly understood to have continued into the 1960s and '70s, and it was not without tragedy. By the time the thalidomide scandal broke, many thousands of babies had been injured *in utero* when their mothers were given thalidomide – a drug developed in the 1950s – to treat nausea in pregnancy. In the US, the Food and Drug Administration (FDA) had not formally granted authority for sale of the drug, but it did enter the country and it was actively sold elsewhere, including in the UK and wider European nations.[11] In response to the thalidomide crisis, state regulations around drug safety were ramped-up. In the US, the performance of clinical research trials became a prerequisite for FDA approval of pharmaceuticals.[12] This, it would seem, came to be interpreted as the use of RCTs.[13]

In Marxist terms, there is distinct logic to the state involving itself in regulation of this kind. As capitalists are by definition in competition with one another, it follows that no individual capitalist or single group of them is capable of articulating their general and shared interests. That role of ensuring and protecting the conditions allowing for accumulation is conferred to what Mandel describes as a 'special apparatus': namely, the state.[14] In seeking to regulate drugs via an approval process, the capitalist state is on the one hand providing the public with a level of protection from the potential dangers of a pharmaceutical industry (that is driven by the making of profit, rather than entirely health concerns), whilst decidedly *not* dismantling either that industry or its profit motive. RCT results inform pharmaceutical approvals and therefore regulatory decision-making, which is not to deny that research studies sponsored by the manufacturing company of a product appear more likely to generate favourable results regarding the desired effects of that product, than do those studies that are otherwise sponsored.[15]

When Cochrane called upon his medical colleagues to develop and use evidence, he was aware that RCTs can be more difficult to conduct in some areas of healthcare than others. 'It's much easier to randomise pills than operations,' he observed.[16] This was not to be viewed as a deterrent. In pointing towards the various 'expensive innovations'[17] that obstetrics had introduced into routine antenatal, birth and postnatal care, Cochrane was underlining that technologies, as well as pharmaceuticals more specifically, are open to investigation via RCTs. As he was addressing doctors rather than device manufacturers in his 1978 speech, Cochrane was not directly holding the latter to account for their products. He was nonetheless indicating that doctors should think twice – or more precisely carry out rigorous research – before introducing such developments into their practice. As perinatologist Marsden Wagner argued some years later, 'scientific evaluation of birth technology has come as an afterthought, not a prerequisite for its application.'[18] He indicated that commercial interests had considerable control over the assessment of birthing technologies, and whilst doctors often conducted research, their relationships with manufacturers were not always transparent.[19]

As the era of late capitalism ushered in a proliferation of screens, computers, large online data banks, information retrieval systems and virtual worlds of communication, these developments were used to facilitate the conducting of research, but they were also important for the sharing of results. Health professionals' access to desktop computers increased, enabling them to stay abreast of new research and clinical trials:[20] 'Remote electronic access to research reports provided an easy path to a massive archive of information, replacing the need to visit a physical library with printed publications.'[21] The early founders of the movement for clinical evidence made effective use of information technology as they began to develop what later became known as the Cochrane Library: 'a collection of databases that contain high-quality, independent evidence to inform healthcare decision-making'.[22] At the time of writing this book, the Cochrane Library reports that its database containing bibliographic records of RCTs contains over two million of these records.[23] Many of these relate specifically to pregnancy and childbirth. The Cochrane Library also includes a database of systematic reviews – that is, reviews published through Cochrane which discuss all the existing evidence that meets predetermined criteria, on a particular topic.[24]

However laudable the early calls for evidence-based medicine were, they have also been criticised for merging rather uncomfortably with an increasingly prevalent neoliberal agenda. It was just the year after Cochrane described obstetrics and gynaecology worthy of a 'wooden spoon' award for practice evaluation, that Margaret Thatcher came to power. In this context, Cochrane has been described as amongst the 'early voices in a neoliberal chorus, questioning all traditional claims of medical professionalism'.[25] In his book *Effectiveness and Efficiency: Random Reflections on Health Services*, he depicted himself as supportive of the national health system not least on social-justice grounds, whilst also having reservations about the state of the service: '… I view the NHS now rather as one would a favourite child who is showing marked delinquent tendencies.'[26] Cochrane was concerned about what he called 'the input/output problem': that more money was flowing into the service than could be justified by the (health) returns.[27] He saw the use of scientific research, particularly Randomised Controlled Trials, as integral to the means by which more 'value for money' could potentially be ascertained; with precise understanding of which 'cures' work, spending might be more appropriately focused. Given that even a publicly funded health service within a capitalist society purchases goods made in surplus-value producing conditions, often from large capitalist companies (monopolies even), the use of costly products that do not entirely meet health needs is not entirely surprising. Yet a neoliberal approach does not challenge capitalism, and Cochrane was certainly not a Marxist. He has been criticised, by a doctor who described himself as one of Cochrane's 'more wayward apprentices', for viewing medical care as essentially a production process within which basic assumptions of mainstream classical economic theory (one might say balancing of input and output) are considered relevant.[28] Those presuppositions, argued his radical apprentice Dr Julian Tudor Hart, 'have neither explained nor predicted the behaviour of any real economy in 200 years' – it would be surprising if they could adequately account for contemporary healthcare.[29] Marxists indeed emphasise that 'input' and 'output' in a capitalist labour process will never balance for the working class; it is precisely because the people produce far more than they are able to take out, that profit is systematically reaped and the system is crisis ridden. That was not an insight which was at the foreground of Cochrane's – or many other people's – consideration during the years of neoliberalism when evidence-based medicine was rising in popularity.

By the time the evidence-based healthcare movement was gaining ground in the 1990s, a range of circumstances had emerged, converged and consolidated, supporting that to happen. Birth had moved largely into hospital-based services, and a new range of equipment and apparatus was increasingly available on the global market for purchase and use in those environments. In calling for evidence, doctors, health workers and later activist groups were demanding proof that the emergent procedures actually had effects that were hoped for and anticipated. If capital had accumulated for the pharmaceutical and medical-tech companies, this was also the era in which states were beginning to constrain public-sector spending and in a somewhat ironic twist of fate, it appeared that 'evidence' could be called upon in alignment with that process. In comparison to other areas of medicine and surgery, 'evidence' was perhaps of particular significance for obstetrics and gynaecology because the 'patients' were primarily women. As has been noted by feminist sociologist of birth Barbara Katz Rothman, 'We were, I can assure you, no longer patient.'[30] Calls for evidence became integral to feminist demands that obstetrics – then still a primarily male profession – cease to impose its own traditions, preferences and convenience upon entire populations of childbearing people. By the end of the twentieth century, *evidence* was being widely advocated within health and pregnancy care contexts, and from a range of not entirely convergent perspectives.

HIERARCHIES, RCTS AND EXPERIMENTS

It may well be that RCTs initially gained prominence because of their significance to the pharmaceutical industry, but in time they became crucial to the evidence-based medicine movement more generally. In that latter context, a 'hierarchy of evidence' was established in which knowledge derived in different ways was ranked according to its reliability and trustworthiness to inform clinical decision-making, and at the lofty apex of the pyramid was situated the Randomised Controlled Trial.[31] Such phenomena as small sample size were acknowledged to limit the possibilities offered by RCTs, but this form of study came to be widely viewed as exemplary of what science had to offer in evaluating clinical treatments or interventions. Ranked below the RCT within the hierarchy were other forms of evidence. These included, but were not limited to, evidence derived from cohort studies (which involve, for instance, observation of the health of people in cohorts over time), and case-control studies (in which a group of people with a specific health outcome, and a control-group, are identified, and focus might be on looking back to identify factors associated with the health outcome under investigation).[32]

RCTs do have distinct methodological strengths which are seen to reduce 'bias' in epidemiological terms. The fact that randomisation is intrinsic to the study design is understood to be important in this respect. In simple terms, within an RCT, research participants are allocated via a randomisation scheme to either an intervention group or a control group, and this helps to ensure that the population of those groups do not differ in systematic ways.[33] For instance, if people in the intervention group were healthier than those in the control group, it might be pre-existing health status rather than the intervention itself which affects the outcomes for that group. Processes of randomisation help to guard against eventualities such as that. Within RCTs there is often the capacity for research participants and a range of other involved parties – the researchers, for example – to be masked (sometimes referred to as 'blinded').[34] This means that they are not made aware of which 'treatment' they, or the different groups within the study, are receiving (a drug or a placebo, for example). In that way, the extent to which people's own preferences or assumptions regarding specific treatments might affect their behaviour – and therefore the findings of a trial – are seen to be minimised. In short, 'With subjects properly randomized and with investigators blind to which is the experimental group and which is the control group, it provides the best way to determine whether something works and allows bias of various kinds to be controlled to a large extent.'[35] Integral to the positioning of RCTs as the gold-standard research design were, therefore, a number of broader presuppositions regarding what constitutes good science.

Unlike other forms of clinical evidence such as cohort studies, RCTs also involve the staging of an experiment. Marxist philosopher of science Alfred Sohn-Rethel contends that the modern experimental method is particularly well suited to knowledge production within capitalist conditions.[36] He emphasised that in modern science, experiments do not involve the investigation of phenomena in the contexts in which those phenomena usually occur. Instead, a set of well-defined and controlled conditions are developed and a phenomenon is explored within that experimental milieu. Depending on the outcome of such experiments, a 'law of recurrent events' might be established which is then used and applied in broader contexts.[37] For Sohn-Rethel, such an approach to the generation of knowledge is entirely congruent with the capitalist mode of production in which labourers are not the primary people organising, planning and controlling their work processes; nor can they be trusted by the bourgeoisie to do so. Instead of relying upon the understanding of workers who carry out a job every day, knowledge is obtained in experimental conditions and then used by the capitalist class for what Sohn-Rethel called 'technological application' within the capitalist workplace.[38] Sohn-Rethel was not writing specifically about RCTs. Indeed, his reflections on experiments are integral to his discussion of the work of Galileo.[39] Nonetheless there is at least one striking resonance. Contemporary philosopher of science Nancy Cartwright notes that the results of RCTs are 'often treated as if the results can be exported in the way that Galileo's results could'.[40] And that may be the case, even if such exportation is not actually possible. When the results of an RCT are highly dependent upon environmental factors such as the skills of birth workers, or the specific ways in which a health system is structured, the 'external validity' of a study – broadly speaking the extent to which the findings of a study are generalisable to people or environments beyond the confines of the study itself – can be quite limited.

RCTs can also be expensive to carry out, particularly on a large scale, and it may be easier to conduct RCTs which last for a short period of time. Yet sizeable, long-duration studies may be precisely what is required to ensure that long-term negative effects of particular treatments are identified. It has been noted, for instance, that 'RCTs may be of limited value in the assessment of harms of interventions because RCTs are frequently small and/or of too short duration for uncommon harms or longer-term harms to be detected.'[41] This is an important observation. It is one thing to focus upon the effects (positive or negative) of treatments which doctors and nurses see during a person's hospital stay, but quite another to consider those which people might be living with and dealing with years after they have been discharged from hospital. Moreover, however well conducted an RCT may be, it does not and cannot provide all the information needed to ascertain exactly what will work for an individual person when *they* are in the midst of having a baby. In the discussion which follows, I consider the relevance of such issues with particular reference to an RCT which is well known within contemporary birth care contexts: the so-called 'Term Breech Trial'.[42]

THE TERM BREECH TRIAL

Babies who are in a breech position *in utero* are often described as being 'butt first'. They have their 'breech' – to use an archaic English word – pointing downwards, towards the opening of the womb. Many foetuses will move into a breech position at some point, yet when a pregnancy reaches 'term' or 'full-term' (often defined as 37 or more weeks of gestation, with an 'estimated due date' usually being set at around 40 weeks of pregnancy), the majority are 'head down'. The authors of the 'Term Breech Trial' wrote that around 3–4 per cent of babies are in a breech position when a pregnancy reaches term.[43] I acknowledge that there are recommendations regarding redefinition of what 'term' means in the US.[44] However, in this chapter, I use the word 'term' in reference to pregnancies of 37 or more weeks' gestation as that is how the word was defined in the RCT under discussion.

Vaginal breech births are broadly considered more complicated than when the baby is in a head-down position, as the largest part of the baby's anatomy (the head) is born after the rest of the body. Challenges can arise, for instance, from compression of the cord – through which the baby's oxygen supply travels – towards the end of a birth.[45] Around the end of the twentieth century, concern was being expressed in medical circles (to some extent influenced by emergent research[46]) that the planning of a caesarean may be the safest way to approach breech births at term. In that context, the 'Term Breech Trial' was devised. The principal investigators wrote that they 'wished to give the option of vaginal breech birth its best, and perhaps last, chance to be proven a reasonable method of delivery'.[47] It was a bold, if rather ominous, claim to make.

The Term Breech Trial was a large Randomised Controlled Trial in which data was collected on over 2,000 women, across 121 centres (hospitals/maternity units, etc.) in 26 countries. Research participants in the trial were required to have a breech pregnancy of one baby at term, and for that baby to be in either a frank or a complete breech position (in other words with legs pointing straight upwards, or with both knees bent and feet close to the buttocks). Participants were randomly allocated to either a planned caesarean section or a planned vaginal birth group.[48] The findings of the study were published in 2000.[49] It was reported that in cases where a caesarean section had been planned, there were significantly lower rates of 'perinatal mortality, neonatal mortality, or serious neonatal morbidity' (broadly speaking, complications for the foetuses/neonates) than was the case when a vaginal birth was planned.[50] Of babies whose birth was planned by caesarean, 1.6 per cent were reported to have had such outcomes, compared to 5 per cent of those who were allocated to the planned vaginal birth group. In terms of mortality and serious morbidity for mothers, the authors reported that there were no significant differences between the two wings of the study. According to their own interpretation of the data, 'Planned caesarean section is better than planned vaginal birth for the term fetus in the breech presentation; serious maternal complications are similar between the groups.'[51]

There have been many critiques of the Term Breech Trial. These having included concerns that research participants did not fit the criteria for inclusion in the trial, and that of the 16 cases involving stillbirths/neonatal mortality, two of those deaths were acknowledged by the primary investigators as probably occurring before the mother was recruited to the study.[52] For the purposes of the discussion at hand, however, the birthing of a baby in a breech position is very different from the swallowing of a drug or the administration of a pharmaceutical product – and as Cochrane had himself acknowledged, it is far easier to 'randomise pills' than it is to randomise many other aspects of healthcare. It is entirely unethical to randomise a research participant to a strictly vaginal breech birth group because during the course of their labour, it may become apparent that they need a caesarean section. Therefore, the 'Term Breech Trial' was analysed on the basis of what is called *intention to treat*. That is to say, people were allocated either to the group of people *intended* to have a caesarean section, or to the group *intended* to have a vaginal birth. Many, particularly in the latter group, did not end up with the mode of birth that was initially intended. This is a legitimate form of RCT analysis – although not without its challenges – but the relevance of the fact that the birthing of babies in a breech presentation is very different to the taking or administering a pill, extends well beyond that.

Providing safe clinical support for someone who is having a vaginal breech birth, has been described as a process requiring considerable knowledge, clinical judgement and discernment.[53] If a doctor or midwife is attending a breech birth, the quality of their skills is important. Drawing upon Marxist terminology, it might be argued that the specific nature or character of the *living labour* of the birth attendant can make a considerable difference to what happens during, and therefore the outcomes of, that birth. It was noted by a doctor who commented on the trial, that ensuring consistent quality of clinical practice across midwives and doctors within a study involving 121 globally participating centres can be incredibly difficult – if it is possible at all.[54] He described the Term Breech Trial protocol outlining how labours were to be managed within that study as relatively 'simple'[55] and that may have been necessary to account for the fact that there were many birth workers involved in the study, and there are many differences in how clinicians support and attend breech births. Yet in its apparent simplicity, the protocol appears to have omitted specifications that would have enhanced safety. For instance, it was suggested that not many obstetricians who work in locations where vaginal breech birth is safely supported, would have found the maximum timescale specified for the second stage of labour within the RCT acceptable.[56] Concern has also been expressed regarding the ways in which the use of pharmaceuticals to induce and accelerate labour was permitted within the study.[57]

RCTs can be very useful for evaluating what obstetrician Murray Enkin refers to as the '(average) relative effects of alternative forms of care … where the form of care used is the principal cause of the outcome found'.[58] As philosopher of science Nancy Cartwright explains, 'RCTs can measure the (average) contribution a treatment makes – if there is a stable contribution to be measured.'[59] This is important information to obtain (or it can be), but it is decidedly *not* the same as establishing what the effect of a particular treatment will be for a particular person who is pregnant and who is contemplating whether a particular 'intervention' might work well for them or not. In everyday life, people are seldom, if ever, *average*: they have a range of physical, social, cultural and unique personal characteristics which may well contribute to how a particular treatment effects *them*. The authors of a recent paper in the *Social Science and Medicine* journal, explain this in the following way:

> If your physician tells you that she endorses evidence-based medicine, and that the drug will work for you because an RCT has shown that 'it works', it is time to find a physician who knows that you and the average are not the same.[60]

In this respect, the results of RCTs require careful interpretation when they are used to inform the treatment of individual people. In the case of the Term Breech Trial, this issue was further complicated by the aforementioned variability occurring across at least one of the 'treatments'. Amongst those people who were randomised to the planned vaginal birth group, some had their labour accelerated with pharmaceutical oxytocin and others did not; some people had their labours induced, whilst others didn't.[61] The authors of the Term Breech Trial stated that women within the trial 'having a vaginal breech delivery had an experienced clinician at the birth',[62] whilst also expressing awareness, within the same article, that the definitions used within the trial of 'vaginal breech-delivery experience' may not have been 'true measures of experience'.[63] One prominent obstetrician commentator argued that in the case of the Term Breech Trial – due to issues such as those outlined above – the researchers were reporting on 'an average level of care'.[64] That is to say, the Term Breech Trial analysis was indicating 'an average level of care, in an average population'.[65] Reporting on average care may not be entirely problematic, in that many breech births may indeed take place in conditions that are rather average – so too do caesarean sections – but if *quality*, rather than *average*, birth care is being aimed towards, the Term Breech Trial fell considerably short of constituting 'the definitive study of vaginal breech delivery'.[66] This particular commentator was concerned that in units or locations where the skills of birth workers in attending vaginal breech births are of a high quality – above the average – the conclusions of the Term Breech Trial would simply not be valid.

Yet the results of RCTs – and experiments more generally – are often assumed to be relevant beyond the experimental context, and the Term Breech Trial was certainly no exception in that respect. Hospital practice regarding breech births changed rapidly following the publication of that particular RCT. This was the case to the extent that many would agree with the comment that 'Rarely in medical history have the results of a single research project so profoundly and so ubiquitously changed medical practice, as in the case of this publication.'[67] After the trial was published, 19 out of 20 Canadian maternity hospitals reported a rise in the proportion of breech births taking place by caesarean, and 65 per cent reported that rates increased 'markedly'.[68] In the Netherlands, the caesarean rate for babies presenting by the breech at term rose from 50 to 80 per cent within two months of the trial's publication.[69] More recently, rates of caesarean section for breech births are reported to be well above 86 per cent in Australia, Scotland, England and Wales.[70] It is even documented that in the UK the caesarean rate for babies who are persistently breech, is around 96 per cent.[71] Vaginal breech births have been described as 'an exceedingly rare event' in the US.[72]

The results of the Term Breech Trial were doubtless important in informing subsequent developments. But they did not act alone. Indeed, if it is useful to avoid the fetishisation of technology, it may also be exigent to avoid attributing excessive power to a single RCT. Declining rates of vaginal breech birth were already underway prior to the publication of the Term Breech Trial.[73] On the basis of data obtained from the trial from countries with low rates of perinatal death, and additional information from Canada, it was estimated that planned vaginal birth was more financially costly than planned c-section when a baby was in a breech position at term in pregnancies involving a single baby (rather than twins, etc).[74] It seems quite possible that even prior to the Term Breech Trial, rates of planned caesareans for breech births were rising for economic and financially related reasons, at least in parts of the Global North. The majority of legal cases around birth which pertain to caesarean section involve allegations of tardiness or of failure to conduct the surgery, as opposed to performance of an unnecessary operation.[75] Given such a combination of circumstances, perhaps it is not surprising that 'the conclusions of the Term Breech Trial are perceived today by many obstetricians as a badly needed set of arguments for PCS [primary caesarean section], which they would have preferred anyway.'[76]

Obstetricians need considerable skill to perform a caesarean section but more still, it would seem, to safely support a vaginal breech birth. In the words of a commenting Professor of Obstetrics and Gynaecology, 'learning how to do a cesarean section is a lot easier than learning how to conduct a vaginal breech birth.'[77] This may help to explain the rapid uptake of the conclusions of the Term Breech Trial team. As a consultant obstetrician in Ireland commented, 'unlike other clinical trials, the findings have been enthusiastically embraced by clinicians, perhaps because for obstetricians elective caesarean section is an easier option than vaginal breech delivery.'[78] Opportunities for obstetricians and midwives to develop and maintain skills in safely supporting vaginal breech births may have been declining prior to the Term Breech Trial, but they have since dropped further. The cycle is self-perpetuating: rising rates of caesarean for babies in a breech position at term reduce the opportunities for birth workers to learn, develop and maintain practical knowledge, skills and experience in supporting vaginal breech birthing. Writing seven years after the trial, a Canadian commentator observed that 'a new generation of specialist obstetricians' had emerged who were, and perhaps for the first time in obstetric history, without 'the skill and confidence to attend even the most straightforward vaginal breech birth'.[79]

The metamorphosis of workforce skills is not unique to pregnancy and birth-care contexts. Marx was acutely aware that as capital accumulates, technologies develop and divisions of labour shift, such that the day-to-day activities of workers also change. He quoted the words of Andrew Ure, who was a chemist of the time, regarding the substituting of 'one description of human labour for another', and that included 'the less skilled for the more skilled'.[80] Over a century later, Harry Braverman argued that as capitalism develops 'the very concept of skill becomes degraded.'[81] Workers may have historically spent years of their life in apprenticeship situations developing and learning specific forms of work and craft, and in late twentieth-century capitalism, skill may be accredited by a certificate which is completed within a few days – hours even. Workers lose abilities they could have previously spent years perfecting, and as scientific and technological developments are introduced into labour processes, people also lose in-depth understanding of much of the work in which they are involved. In the context of a caesarean birth, surgeons focus upon surgery, anaesthetists upon anaesthetics, neonatologists, and other workers – nurses or midwives – have different tasks again. The divisions of labour are considerable, and vary from one locality to another. I'm not entirely convinced that people become *less* skilled as such developments unfold, but people do lose skills in certain areas. The honing of skills in the facilitation of caesarean sections has certainly corresponded with a loss of skills in supporting vaginal breech birthing.

Research developments after the publication of the Term Breech Trial have proven insufficient to reverse this trend. Following the publication of the Term Breech Trial, a follow-up study was conducted which raised questions around whether the shift towards caesarean section was as necessary as proponents of the Term Breech Trial had initially suggested it was. This research collected information, two years later, on a sub-group of infants who had been part of the Term Breech Trial and found that by that time, the incidence of death and neurodevelopmental delay for those who had been in the planned caesarean group and the planned vaginal birth group were similar (3.1 and 2.8 per cent respectively).[82] Any prevailing assumptions that neonatal morbidity had predicted future outcomes of the neurological kind, were thereby called into question.[83] If abdominal births are being carried out for health reasons, it would be anticipated that long-term health is taken into account. It is, after all, *that* which babies and adults live with after – perhaps for decades after – they are discharged from maternity hospitals. In addition to this, the 2006 findings of a large observation study in France and Belgium found that within that context, neonatal outcomes for term breech babies did not differ significantly whether it had been planned for the infant to be born vaginally or via caesarean section.[84] The authors concluded that 'In places where planned vaginal delivery is a common practice and when strict criteria are met before and during labor, planned vaginal delivery of singleton fetuses in breech presentation at term remains a safe option that can be offered to women.'[85] Arguably by then, however, the die had been cast. A further survey conducted in Canada indicated that hospitals were far more likely to foster a protocol requiring caesarean for breech births after the Term Breech Trial was published, than to change such a policy after the follow-up study came out.[86] The authors noted a lack of localities where vaginal breech birthing was well provided for, validated and studied, and where the skills to safely support those births were being maintained and developed. Canada is far from alone in that respect.

Rapid transformation of workforce knowledge and skill is an ongoing feature of capitalism, but it has particular effects in pregnancy care contexts. So long as people gestate, it seems to me that vaginal breech births will continue to happen. Many people *do* want to birth in this way, and babies can assume a breech position without that being apparent until they are just about to be born. In this respect, loss of birth-worker skills around supporting different forms of birthing creates considerable problems – and the kinds of problems that simply do not arise when skills change in other areas of the economy where people are working primarily with inanimate objects. One doctors explains: 'The anxiety and atmosphere caused by a quickly progressing breech in labour on a delivery unit is unique as it essentially represents a normal physiological process causing what is now considered a medical emergency.'[87] There are various examples of women dying because a caesarean was considered the only viable course of action, but with skilled practitioners, a vaginal breech birth may have been quite possible.[88] For pregnant people who today *do* want to plan a vaginal breech birth, it is increasingly difficult for them to find a midwife or doctor who is experienced, skilled and willing to support them in that. These people speak of 'stress, anger, fear and injustice' regarding the situations they face.[89] Responsibility might be placed with the Term Breech Trial – as it is widely viewed as having transformed practice around breech birthing across the world. Yet that RCT can also be read as an effect and iteration of dynamics and relationships, integral to capitalism, in which technological 'solutions' are prioritised over investment into the complexities and diversities of labour needed to support safe birthing. A range of doctors and midwives have been working hard to revive, develop and nourish clinician skills and experience in attending breech births.[90] However, the extent to which they will be successful in the contemporary climate remains to be seen.

Vaginal breech births are not advisable for all babies in a breech position at term – some it would seem fare better than others – but pressures towards universal caesarean section are not acceptable. Today, there is considerable concern regarding opportunities for breech birth in the Global South. In countries where birth rates are comparatively high, and in which safe surgical facilities are few and far between, the dangers to people of having a caesarean (especially if not needed) are particularly elevated. Focused upon short-term indicators (as RCTs tend to be), the Term Breech Trial did not measure the likelihood and effects of scar rupture in a future pregnancy for people who had previously had a planned caesarean for breech presentation and where there are few emergency health facilities available. In the words of a physician in The Gambia writing a letter to a major medical journal at the time, 'Skills for vaginal delivering of breech babies must not be lost, and doctors the world over must continue to disagree with a policy of inflicting caesarean scars because it suits the practice of the richer nations.'[91] Concerns of this kind remain valid to this day. In 2023, Consultant Obstetrician and Gynaecologist Sabrina Das expressed a related sentiment, drawing upon the language of risk to do so. 'Research findings in high-income settings', she argues, 'cannot be universally applied to low-income settings as the risk-benefit ratio for maternal and neonatal health is dependent on cultural and societal contexts.'[92] Such a ratio is dependent, I suggest, upon the operations and local determinations of an intensely racialised and global capitalism. Das herself emphasises the need to invest in training for people attending vaginal breech births, *as well as* ensuring that safe caesareans are available when needed. I agree.

COLLAPSE OF THE GOLD STANDARD?

In late twentieth-century capitalism, RCTs were designated the 'gold standard' for research on the effects of medical interventions. Yet knowledge derived from RCTs, like any form of knowledge, has limitations and perhaps this is now increasingly acknowledged.[93] As two influential commentators recently noted:

> Experiments are sometimes the best that can be done, but they are often not. Hierarchies that privilege RCTs over any other evidence irrespective of context or quality are indefensible and can lead to harmful policies. Different methods have different relative advantages and disadvantages.[94]

RCTs are often not well suited to ascertaining the long-term and inadvertent effects of particular interventions; due to issues of so-called 'external validity', the results will not necessarily be replicable in clinical environments beyond the study context. Nonetheless, to this day birth workers – including doctors – often have to work hard to prove that specific RCT findings will *not* be replicable within their own workplaces. For example, the publication of a 2018 US trial regarding induction of labour was followed by a number of articles and studies from across the world in which authors worked hard to explain and demonstrate that the RCT was *not* relevant within the contexts and population that *they* work with.[95] Recent research indicates that use of induction of labour (in circumstances related to the original trial) did rise in various US hospitals after the publication of the RCT, although not necessarily with the anticipated effects.[96]

Although RCTs rose to prominence within the context of particular late-capitalist developments, such as the burgeoning of the pharmaceutical industry, there have been many developments since then. For instance, work has been ongoing for some time in developing and enhancing RCT methodology, e.g., in supporting 'complex interventions' (those involving many threads of interactions) to be evaluated using RCTs.[97] Given the large amount of evidence now being produced, and the premise that scientific knowledge progresses on the basis of cumulation, proponents of evidence-based medicine often emphasise the importance of systematic reviews of existing evidence and occasionally these reviews have been placed above RCTs in hierarchies of evidence.[98] This latter move is not entirely unproblematic, as it suggests that systematic reviews constitute evidence in their own right rather than summaries of already existing evidence. Indicating the diversity of evidence that is today available and necessary for particular questions with clinical relevance to be answered, some systematic reviews now incorporate consideration of non-RCT research, such as case-control studies, cohort studies, etc.[99] The GRADE (Grading of Recommendations, Assessment, Development, and Evaluations) framework has been developed – a tool which facilitates the grading of evidence according to quality and supports the making of recommendations for clinical practice.[100] Yet even if a particular medical intervention is strongly recommended in a specific context, there are no guarantees that it will actually work for or be acceptable to a particular person within their own given set of social and other circumstances. If pregnant people are to be acknowledged as more than 'vessels' for the safe delivery of a baby, this is important. Early advocates described evidence-based medicine as 'the conscientious, explicit, and judicious use of current best evidence in making decisions about the care of individual patients', and they indicated that such an approach also requires 'thoughtful identification and compassionate use of individual patients' predicaments, rights and preferences'.[101] Whilst I'm keen to resist the somewhat atomised view of pregnant people as discrete isolated individuals in one-to-one dialogue with individual clinicians (far more comes into childbirth decision-making than that), aspects of such an analysis remain relevant to this day. Evidence derived from the health sciences – whether from RCTs or not – is insufficient to develop birth care that is safe and nourishing for all.

In addition to this, much contemporary health-science research is focused upon establishing the effects of discrete (often commodified) 'interventions', and is therefore ill-suited to exploring the complex webs of social relations and dynamics that contribute to such products being developed and presented for the market in the first place. As Marxist sociologists of medicine have long indicated, in capitalism the focus of medicine is the treatment of individuals through specific clinical interventions such as pharmaceuticals, rather than upon the social relations which so often give rise to and/or exacerbate ill health and might therefore need to be changed to maximise health. Intimately related is Sheryl Burt Ruzek's point that so much research within the medical science literature is focused upon what she calls 'capital-intensive products'.[102] Research indicating the benefits of midwifery continuity of care, for instance, tends not to receive the same attention and traction as that which points in the direction of heavily technologised obstetric interventions, and there is now analysis demonstrating that many clinical guidelines are *not* based upon high-quality evidence anyway.[103] Robbie Davis-Floyd notes that where birth analysts have often highlighted an 'evidence-practice gap', there is now an 'evidence-discourse-practice gap': doctors speak of and emphasise the importance of evidence, whilst simultaneously overlooking and discounting evidence that is not in accordance with the prevailing norms of 'technomedical treatment' and practice.[104] In order to grapple with *why* such issues haunt so many pregnancy and birth-care services, I find it useful to remind myself of the ongoing allure and significance of technological fetishism within contemporary capitalism; I find it helpful to reflect again on the continuing pull and traction of the largely invisible social relations of capitalism upon people's (including health professionals') lives, practices and the ways in which we make sense of the world – and of course birth.

Fredric Jameson indicates that the totality of capitalism is so vast and burgeoning, that no single form of knowledge is adequate to understand its articulations in people's lives. He goes so far as to suggest that all attempts to represent capitalism are themselves 'a mixture of approaches', and that such combinations signal 'the multiple perspectives from which one must approach such a totality' – none being entirely exhaustive.[105] That is no excuse, he contends, to avoid attempting the work of such representation but instead an indication of the need to redouble energies in this regard and to engage dialectically with the incompatibilities and contradictions encountered. I think similarly about childbearing, and not least childbearing within the context of the growing, shifting, totality that is global capitalism with all of its inequities and capacities to draw diverse peoples into its webs of often illusive interconnection. As people give birth to new generations today, knowledge of the latest findings of well-conducted RCTs can be informative, as can that of cohort studies and other observational analyses. Understanding of physiology and anatomy is important too, as might be knowledge of legal restrictions or hospital practices, for example – not to mention knowledge of the intensely social relations which lurk beneath those. But childbearing can also be acutely unsafe if it is not grounded in the distinct needs of childbearing people as they live and birth within communities integral to themselves. Midwives, doctors, etc., frequently *do not know* the details of those, and sometimes those needs may be considerably at odds with the demands that hospitals and employers place upon health workers, or the assumptions that birth workers themselves make and hold. Perhaps it is not surprising therefore, that as calls for evidence rose to prominence within pregnancy-care contexts towards the end of the twentieth century, so too did calls for pregnant people – women tended to be the word that was used – to actively *choose* what happens to them whilst they are in labour. Choice is the focus of the next chapter, and of course it is choice as situated within the context of a rapidly expanding mode of production.

6

Freedom of Choice?

Childbearing people are not new to making decisions about how they approach their pregnancies and childbirth. At different points and places in history, women have called upon various people to be with them as they labour: family, neighbours, midwives, doulas, healers and/or doctors, etc. They have opted to birth in particular locations, and have decided to use certain birthing positions rather than others. As herbs and plants have been used in pregnancy and birthing for centuries, it seems very likely that child-bearing people have been actively involved in determining which remedies to use given their own circumstances or ailments. This is not to deny that circumstance, culture, shared decision-making and at times coercion have historically shaped the contours of birthing, but it would be naïve to assume that pregnant people have not been agents in their own parturient processes. Nevertheless, it was not until the latter decades of the twentieth century that the notion of choice emerged as a pre-eminent principle – a political injunction even – regarding childbirth. Around that time, resources, leaflets and information began to be produced presenting an array of choices people might encounter as they navigated the perinatal services. In some areas, there were specific midwives or doctors to choose from. In others, one could plan to birth in a particular hospital rather than another, in an out-of-hospital birth centre, or at home supported by experienced birth workers. Hospitals started to offer a range of pharmacological pain-relief options including inhalation analgesia ('gas and air'), opioids and epidural analgesia. Various genetic tests, screening and diagnostic options became available in pregnancy, and in this prenatal context, choice has been described as 'a cardinal theme'.[1] Birth activists have often been at the forefront of emphasising the importance of choice in pregnancy and childbirth – lobbying, campaigning, educating and producing information on different options and forms of care.

A range of social and political-economic dynamics facilitated the emergence of choice as a prevalent demand and expectation around childbirth in the late twentieth century, and a key purpose of this chapter is to trace and highlight that 'coming-together' – that amalgamation – of diverse processes. By this account, celebrations of 'choice in childbirth' arose as both a product of and political response to diverse aspects of an expanding capitalism as it transitioned into the neoliberal era. Yet despite the weight and significance attributed to choice in pregnancy, birth is not an arena in which 'freedom of choice' reigns entirely uncircumscribed. Through the chapters of this book, I have indicated various ways in which birthing options are shaped and constrained in the context of capitalism. Formulations of risk, the widespread deployment of technologies not least to accelerate labour processes, and ongoing loss of skills on the part of doctors and midwives, are influential in this respect. Given such a backdrop, perhaps it is unsurprising that Marx's words on history resonate through the discussion which follows. People 'make their own history', he wrote, 'But they do not make it just as they please in circumstances they choose for themselves; rather they make it in present circumstances, given and inherited.'[2] Similar can be said of birthing. People make decisions which can profoundly influence the ways in which birth happens. Yet they neither have complete control over birthing, nor do they make choices in conditions they would necessarily choose for themselves. Such themes are developed in this chapter through consideration of aspects of childbirth most prevalently associated with decisions made by childbearing people, for example, pain relief, pre-labour caesarean sections and freebirthing (births that are planned to take place without a doctor or midwife present). In addition to that, while choice in contemporary capitalism has been simultaneously venerated and constrained (more so for some social groups than others), capitalism is *also* a mode of production which actively generates crises and disaster situations in which choice is effectively eradicated. Arguably, such precarious conditions will be increasingly prevalent over coming years. In beginning to explore these contradictions, Marx's early work on the human species as capable of 'conscious life-activity' provides a pertinent starting point.

MARX ON 'CONSCIOUS LIFE-ACTIVITY' AND 'SPECIES BEING'

Marx was aware that people make deliberate decisions which impact their physical bodies as well as the external environment in which they live. He saw, for example, that humans must eat and drink to survive, as must other animals, but that for human beings, such activities are far more than biological necessities.[3] As people have the capacity for what he called 'conscious life-activity',[4] these corporeal processes and the resources used – food, plants, etc. – become objects not only of immediate survival but also of such realms of human life as science, theory, art and spirituality. Unlike other animals, insects, or creatures which build nests, dams and honeycombs, as well as hunting for food, humans can deliberately and consciously develop and calculate long-term strategies for staying warm, fed and hydrated even when they do not immediately need to do so – even when they are not under demanding corporeal pressure to ensure their survival. People can also act in accordance with their own elaborately devised plans, and so it is that humans are able to consciously change – 'work-up' – the 'nature' of which they themselves are a part, in ways that are not available to other species.[5] Marx viewed explicitly human activity as involving a degree of freedom from the immediacy of corporeal existence and from the urgency of drives for survival, and in this respect, he used the term 'species being' (prevalent within Hegelian circles at the time) in reference to the human species.[6] In short, a definitive characteristic of the human species is that they have the capacity to render their own species (and other species) the object of their conscious deliberate enquiry *and* of their own conscious life activity. There are indications in Marx's early writing that he viewed such human capacities as superior to those of other species, and that is a premise which sits uncomfortably with many twenty-first-century understandings as we grapple now with the devastating effects of a 'worked-up' environment upon so many non-human (as well as human) entities. Yet key aspects of the early Marx remain acutely relevant today. He understood, for example, that whilst people have the capacity to produce 'beauty' and 'wonderful things', in capitalism the products of their conscious-life activity accrue in the hands of the rich.[7] That is to say, people actively create a world of which they are denied the pleasures and freedoms – and this is acutely alienating.

Marx also considered the making of people to be a decidedly human process. As sketched in Chapter 2 of this book, he described the creation 'of fresh life in procreation' to be a *social* activity which has existed since time began.[8] In *The Economic and Philosophic Manuscripts of 1844*, Marx noted that although other animals bear young, 'drinking, eating, procreating, etc., are also genuinely human functions.'[9] For him, that is the case when those activities are *not* abstracted from other aspects of conscious human activity – when they are *not* constituted purely as ends in their own right. Marx did not elaborate greatly on procreation within the 1844 manuscripts, and later in those writings his musings on procreation pertain to relations between men and women rather than to childbirth per se.[10] Yet deploying this aspect of his work as a theoretical lever, one might contend that when childbirth is *done* by human beings (rather than reflected upon as an abstraction), birthing is *necessarily* infused with social, cultural and scientific contexts which have developed in that historical milieu; it cannot *but* be shaped by the ways in which human activity has already 'worked-up' the world. For instance, I have already indicated that when people engage in conscious activity around parturition, they draw upon pre-existing technologies, upon particular kinds of science, or upon formulations of risk. Yet through much of the twentieth century at least, it has often been assumed to be doctors and clinicians, rather than childbearing people, who make – and *must* make – the conscious, deliberate decisions regarding parturition. Such an understanding was substantially challenged in the latter years of the second millennium, when a chorus of voices publicly heralding and asserting choice for childbearing people began to resonate across public and birthing spaces. This is an historical development which merits further consideration.

CONSOLIDATIONS OF CHOICE

I have fond and quite early memories of political calls for people to have choice in the ways they give birth. As a child, I remember excitedly opening a package of hundreds of pencils for my midwife-activist mother, and inside I found the words 'choice in childbirth' inscribed on the side of them. I'm not quite sure who or what the pencils were for; perhaps they were to be distributed at a conference or to be strategically placed around the birthing unit of the local NHS hospital. I'm guessing it was the early 1980s, and probably before the effects of neoliberalism had really begun to bite – in England at least. I do recall however, that a few of those pencils lay around the house I grew up in for years, mostly by the side of the phone next to the scraps of paper on which my mother would scribble messages to my sister and myself. At the time, the very mention of choice in childbirth had a somewhat novel feel to it, but use of the word 'choice' in relation to birth was not entirely new. In 1760, English midwife Elizabeth Nihell had used the word 'choice' when writing about birth, but she used it to refer to 'nature's own choice' rather than to decisions made by people.[11] She was arguing that 'choice' made by *nature* predisposes women, rather than men, to the art of midwifery. At that time and place in history, struggles over divisions of labour and over who gets to perform the labour of attending births at all, were intensely gendered and rooted in deeply held beliefs regarding the naturalised roles of men and women. In the early decades of the twentieth century, an influential campaigner for twilight sleep contended that in so far as 'the supreme function of childbearing' is concerned, 'every woman should certainly have the choice of saying how she will have her child.'[12] She continued: 'If scopolamin-morphin is safe and insures amnesia, a mother should have the right to demand that her physician employ these drugs, and if he declines to do so she should feel no hesitation whatever in seeking another doctor who will.'[13] Of course twilight sleep was not safe and many people had no access to doctors at all. However, her calls were indicative of a sensibility, at least amongst women of the wealthier classes, that when choosing from a competitive market of obstetric birth attendants, careful deliberation was required. Substantial study would be necessary to investigate how concepts akin to that of 'choice' have been used and articulated around birth in different historical contexts, and such research lies beyond the scope of the present work. That said, when calls for 'choice' in relation to birth began to reach a crescendo around the 1980s, a relatively recent twentieth-century history was being negotiated, built upon and responded to.

By that time the conditions in which the working class were produced had been an object of state concern and involvement for decades, and the political-economic landscape was changing. Drawing upon Nancy Fraser's periodisation, 'state-managed' capitalist regimes had consolidated in core regions of global industrial production after the Great Depression and the Second World War.[14] Around that time, the state had involved itself in such aspects of life as healthcare provision (focused upon ensuring the 'quality' of existent and future labour power), and the role of housewife came to be expected and more highly normalised than before for large (particularly white) sections of the female population. When diverse political struggles – such as civil rights, anti-imperialist and feminist movements – began to mobilise in opposition to the oppressions of the era, women were demanding to make their own decisions over whether they bore and raised children. This was remarkably fertile ground from which political calls for 'Choice!' in relation to childbearing grew. Initially, calls for choice gained traction around the issue of abortion.[15] 'Choice!' was, in short, an injunction that women be supported to live lives that did not entirely revolve around the production and raising of children. Not only were women asserting themselves as capable of making conscious decisions around these issues. To draw upon the terminology of Marx, they were also capable of 'conscious life activity' that did not involve children.

Alongside such developments, the 1960s was a decade in which state involvement in the provision of birth care expanded. The British Perinatal Mortality Survey had recommended that maternity services be extended, and in the UK birth activist group AIMS (Association for Improvements in the Maternity Services) was campaigning for an increase in the number of hospital beds for women who needed to birth in hospital.[16] But at some point in the 1970s, it became apparent that obstetrics had secured a far more universal remit in relation to birth than the organisation had campaigned for. By then, virtually *all* births were taking place in hospitals and rigid clinical regimes, such as those involving routine episiotomies, were increasingly normalised. As hierarchical staffing structures and clinical paternalism (reflecting nuclear family structures) governed birth service provisions, calls for women to have 'choice in childbirth' were an overtly political response. Any presupposed passivity on the part of childbearing people was being called into question. The assertion was clear: if women are capable of making their own decisions over whether to end a pregnancy, they are *also* capable of making their own conscious deliberate decisions over what is done to their bodies as they birth a baby. That is how I read the words 'choice in childbirth' as they were inscribed on the pencils I excitedly unpacked as a child.

By that point in history, obstetric hospitals were also stocked with the growing range of equipment which, as Cochrane rightly noted, had not been properly evaluated for their clinical effects. The imperative of 'Choice in Childbirth!' was decidedly insufficient if nobody knew nor understood the implications of decisions being made. As paid workers in the Global North were increasingly drawn into jobs involving knowledge production, demands reverberated through activist birth networks that women not only have choice in childbirth, but *informed* choice. By the early 1990s, after intense campaigning by birth activists, the notion of informed choice came to feature in UK parliamentary texts and policy initiatives.[17] Leaflets were produced containing easy-to-read summaries of evidence on topics such as ultrasound scanning, epidurals, possibilities for breech birth and foetal heart monitoring.[18] These texts were aimed at supporting childbearing people to make informed decisions around key aspects of pregnancy care. If, in Marx's terms, the 'conscious life-activity' of paid workers across the world had enabled the production of a range of commodities and medical equipment, childbearing people too could be very deliberately and consciously involved in determining how, and whether, these products were to be used in relation to their own bodies and the infants they were bearing.

Of course, a range of localised dynamics influenced how calls for informed choice unfurled in different jurisdictions. In Aotearoa New Zealand, the Cartwright Inquiry of the 1980s was pivotal.[19] The Inquiry found that women at a major New Zealand teaching hospital had been incorporated into a medical trial on cervical cancer without their informed consent, and some had received inadequate treatment for cervical cancer and died as a result. Vaginal swabs had also been taken from newborn infants in the absence of formal parental agreement. The Women's Health Action organisation which initially instigated the investigation, noted that the inquiry had interconnected with aspects of the feminist health movement and that in time the significance of choice – not least *informed* choice – had come to permeate the New Zealand health sector as a whole.[20]

In this era of intense commodity production and mass consumption of consumer goods, the language of *consumer choice* also entered the lexicon of birth activism. Childbearing people came to be referred to as consumers of pregnancy services, and although it's not a terminology I'm fond of perhaps it is better than talk of *patients* with all the passivity thereby implied. As Barbara Katz Rothman observed, the role of consumer was at that time associated with more power, capacity and decorum than that of the humble patient.[21] In the US, even struggles for access to midwifery care came to be framed in terms of consumer choice. That is not to say that it was a language with which people on low incomes were particularly comfortable: for some, midwifery care was necessity, far more than choice.[22] Midwives had for centuries attended births in working-class areas and within racialised communities. Notwithstanding the virtual eradication of midwifery in the US, to reclaim midwifery through recourse to consumer rights was to draw upon ideological premises endemic to precisely the system which had undermined midwifery in the first place: one might call it racial capitalism.

So it was that towards the end of the twentieth century, as capitalism expanded in unprecedented directions, an array of somewhat variegated demands for choice gathered momentum and converged. Calls for women's choice, informed choice and consumer choice gained traction from disparate directions, and 'choice' consolidated as a prominent demand, an expectation even, in relation to childbirth. It is in this context that I consider choice to have emerged as a 'concrete concept' in relation to childbearing: a 'synthesis of many definitions', to draw upon Marx's words.[23] There were certainly progressive dimensions to the emphasis upon choice which emerged at this time. By various accounts, choice implied autonomy and self-determination on the part of childbearing people who had long been considered passive objects, raw materials even, in conveyor-belt systems of 'care'. In the words of a prominent anthropologist of the time:

> It is not only a matter of 'active birth' and being able to move about – though that is important – but of being an active birth-giver rather than a passive patient. It is basically a question of who accepts the main responsibility, and ultimately with whom the power lies – the obstetrician or you.[24]

However politically necessary and significant their campaigns were, it rapidly became apparent to birth activists that the effects of their endeavours for 'choices in childbirth' were, at best, mixed.

WAS CHOICE THE RIGHT CHOICE?

In a 1998 journal editorial, two UK midwives mused over the trappings of choice. 'Informed choice: Was it the wrong choice?' they asked.[25] These birth workers were particularly concerned that the emphasis being placed upon the facilitation of information-based decision-making was something of a 'red herring'; that it diverted attention away from the fact that much maternity service provision continued to be based upon outdated practices, upon a range of unnecessary constraints and upon hospital policies derived from poor calibre (if any) evidence. They emphasised that the overall *quality* of care needed improvement. The promotion of choice as a mechanism by which people could 'opt out of the routine, suboptimal package of maternity care on offer at their unit' was unfair, an evasion of the issues at stake and unlikely to be successful.[26]

Even if notions of informed choice were to be defended, in the neoliberal climate of the time such enunciations slipped all too easily into acclamations of consumer choice. As midwife Tricia Anderson observed: 'Riding on Margaret Thatcher's wave of the individual taking precedence over society, we began to talk about women as "consumers of maternity care", and as consumers they could exercise choice over what to opt for in childbirth.'[27] I have often wondered whether it was an effect of that particular moment in the emergence of neoliberal capitalism that UK birth activists settled on the language of 'choice' rather than 'decision-making', for their campaigns. The word 'decision' implies more *gravitas*, but is less of a sound-bite perhaps, than 'choice'. Maybe more significantly in historical terms, it does not brim with associations of market freedom. Yet even in capitalism, freedom of the market is a misnomer. Even ardent proponent of capitalism Adam Smith understood that the state (so often depicted in right-wing thought as antithetical to freedom) has a role to play in developing and maintaining publicly advantageous services that would be unprofitable if left to market forces.[28]

Writing as a midwife, Tricia Anderson emphasised that in a supermarket, people choose products based upon such factors such as their availability, visibility on shelves and the shaping of desire through advertising. In so far as childbearing in the UK is concerned, she argued that 'the pregnant woman shopping for her "choices" is led by her local maternity services and what they are able and willing to offer.'[29] Lurking behind that, I would contend, are wider determinants including the staffing, financing and structuring of services, and broader social relations involving the production, marketing and distribution of pharmaceuticals, medical equipment, etc.

Decades after the onset of neoliberalism, the language of choice is still being used in relation to childbirth. In addition to materials produced by hospitals and biomedical service providers, information on pregnancy-related decisions is now sourced through social media, apps, online communities and sources far more widespread than that. It has been suggested that within such unregulated environments, people develop hopes, anticipations and expectancies which may be difficult, if possible at all, to realise.[30] I'm not sure how much has changed over the past two decades in terms of disparity between hopes, aspirations and 'actual' birth outcomes. It is not new to observe that childbearing is seldom an arena in which 'choices' are available or realisable without restriction. As Anderson observed all those years ago, a person may prefer to give birth in a certain way, but there are no guarantees that a particular birth will happen according to predetermined specifications; 'some of us', she wrote, 'for complex reasons – get a 36-hour labour, a trial of forceps [an attempted forceps delivery], an episiotomy, a caesarean and a very cranky baby who won't feed well for weeks.'[31] Anderson was concerned even then, that women were feeling frustrated, disillusioned and disappointed as a result of the prevailing emphasis upon choice. However, and I consider this important, Anderson was *not* arguing that childbearing people have no control in relation to what they do and what happens, in and around childbirth. She was *not* blaming a singular factor, such as a recalcitrant 'nature' or medicalisation, for *why* a particular course of events (e.g., a long labour) might eventuate. She referred to 'complex reasons' for the emergence of particular circumstances, and in so doing was acknowledging that the doing of birth is shaped and determined by many different conditions and relationships. Some of these influences might be corporeal, others social, cultural, or economic, and perhaps at times such classifications obscure more than they reveal. People can certainly make choices and act deliberately in relation to birth, yet such decision-making – and here I return to Marx's insight – is constrained by circumstances which are present and inherited. Moreover, sometimes it is not possible to know exactly *why* particular events happen in certain pregnancies, nor to entirely control for that. In the discussion which follows, I illustrate the historical-determination of childbearing decisions through consideration of so-called 'pain relief' options.

LABOUR PAINS

Pain in birthing has often been considered transhistorical and therefore natural. According to a relatively recent article in the medical literature, 'labour pain is feared and perceived as severe in every culture and ethnic group that has been properly studied.'[32] I have no intention of embarking upon historical research to ascertain the veracity of such a claim, but it does appear that when the pain-relieving effects of chloroform and ether were established in the nineteenth century, some members of the clergy objected to their use in birth on the grounds that God had not intended birth to be painless.[33] By the time twilight sleep became available, there was a clamouring for that form of sedation amongst relatively elite social groups – and not least those who could pay for it. Around the same time and over the decades that followed, a range of twentieth-century practitioners advocated birth preparation and breathing techniques to facilitate or encourage birth without pain. In short, however transhistorical pain in labour may be, approaches to pain and the 'management' of pain in labour vary considerably across historical eras. By the late twentieth century, as neoliberal capitalism rose to prominence, a '"menu" approach to pain in labour' was being adopted in many places of birth.[34] Midwife Nicky Leap wrote of antenatal classes in which people were presented with pain-relief options in a list-like format: 'aromatherapy, water and non-pharmacological methods' might feature towards the top of the menu, followed by offerings such as gas and air, opioids and 'the epidural'.[35]

By that point in the history of capitalism, a sufficiently wide range of products, technologies and procedures were available on the market and/or in birthing spaces that lists of these could indeed be comprised. Given the significance attributed to *evidence* and choice of the *informed* kind, many hospitals would also ensure that a description of the effects (including side-effects) of each list item was available to people choosing from the available options. Yet as Leap was acutely aware, there is more to working with pain in childbirth than menus or lists begin to suggest.

In basic physiological terms, during labour the stretching of muscles and tissue are registered by pain receptors situated at the end of nerve cells. Signals pass along nerve fibres, the spinal cord and to the brain where the 'information' is processed and interpreted. There are various ways in which the transmission of pain signals to the brain can be encouraged or blocked, and a complex range of influences – including physical and psychological – are involved in pain experience.[36] Interactions which effect the levels of beta-endorphins ('endogenous opioids') within the body are significant in this regard.[37] Although some degree of stress is integral to parturition, environments which support a person in labour to feel safe, are understood to encourage optimal levels of these endorphins. A prevailing theme across the literature on pain in childbirth is therefore the positive difference to experiences of pain that ongoing support for a birthing person – the kind of support that helps them to feel safe and unthreatened – can make.[38] Childbearing people's own words reiterate the significance of this. As one explains of a particular birth worker:

> She allowed me to express myself, how I perceived things … I cannot tell you how much she relieved my worries. It was just wonderful … The birth progressed very fast after she came, incredibly faster than before … and I did not suffer such torment as before she came.[39]

In the words of a woman who birthed in an area of London where midwifery care was specifically structured to enable pregnant people to develop a trusting relationship with their birth workers: 'I think it depends on knowing the midwives so well because they do make you feel quite at ease, because if you're scared and you haven't got anyone reassuring you, you're just panicking and it hurts a lot more.'[40] Whatever pain-relief 'choices' may be on offer, highly personalised care from skilled practitioners with whom a birthing person has already developed a familiar and comfortable relationship, is precisely that which is *not* available – and so *cannot* be chosen – in many areas. Indeed, capitalism is not a mode of production characterised by ready and eager investment into labour, particularly into the kinds of labour which build people and communities.

Without paid birth work being well supported, however, the choices of childbearing people are considerably restricted, not least because many contemporary birthing 'options' depend upon that labour being available. As mentioned in Chapter 3, UK-based anaesthetist Dr David Bogod emphasises that it may well *not* be possible for somebody to have an epidural if an anaesthetist is unavailable, or if there are insufficient midwives to ensure safe care involving an epidural.[41] Midwifery shortages, he notes, are 'at the root of so many of the current safety issues facing maternity care in the UK, and we should support our midwifery colleagues in waving this particular banner.'[42] If there is insufficient midwifery staffing to ensure safe care of people with epidurals, serious questions must also be raised regarding the extent to which there is adequate staffing to support childbearing people and their loved ones through labour and more generally. For years, midwives in the UK have been leaving their jobs for reasons related to this: because, for example, they do not feel supported to provide the safe, quality care that they would like to offer.[43]

There are few absolutes in the world of birth, and depending on such factors as staff skills mix and the ways in which birth care is structured, the use of epidurals can have different effects upon staff time and workload. For instance, in some contexts, health professionals may not feel confident supporting people to labour *without* epidurals.[44] In the US, people have been threatened with negative sanctions if they decline epidurals. The researchers of a study in which this was found to be the case, explained that although monitoring of a childbearing person is comparatively intensive after an epidural is in place, that monitoring can be performed at regular intervals. In contrast, 'Caring for an unmedicated woman during birth is arduous, unpredictable, and may take the nurse away from documentation duties for extended periods of time.'[45] They write of there being organisational pressures – imperatives even – for people to have epidurals and of various mechanisms (over and above encouragement or persuasion, and including threat of sanctions) being used to ensure that they do. Within that study, Women of Colour were more likely to be subject to such coercion than were white women. Data obtained on over 2 million childbearing people in the US suggests that around 73 per cent of those who go into labour are receiving epidural (or spinal) analgesia during parturition.[46] Discourses pitched at the level of individual choice are ill-equipped to grapple with the intensely social dynamics which contribute to such a statistic.

Even a Randomised Controlled Trial (RCT) carried out in the UK in 1988 indicated that when 'informed choice' leaflets were distributed to pregnant people and discussed with them by maternity service staff, the pamphlets were presented in such a way as indicating to the childbearing person that 'In any situation there was a "right" choice or course of action.'[47] That course of action may have been 'right' based upon a range of factors including 'research evidence, local circumstances or the individual experiences and skills of those in authority'.[48] Nonetheless, generally speaking, 'women and/or their carers made the "right" choices.' [49] Perhaps that is hardly surprising given that, in the words of the report's authors, 'Problems or "trouble" arose when another choice was made.'[50]

For whatever reasons people arrive at or make particular 'choices', the reification of choice nonetheless leaves childbearing people open to a range of criticisms for the 'choices' they do apparently make. Whilst some speak of being shamed and judged for having an epidural whilst in labour, others undergo criticism for labouring *without* an epidural – and within both contexts, self-blame is often close at hand. Whilst one person notes 'I felt if I hadn't had the epidural maybe it would have gone differently', another indicates 'If only I had the epi[dural] earlier, I would have been able to push him out.'[51] With the most robust evidence and risk-analysis in the world, it is not possible to predict the precise outcomes of particular interventions in a specific set of 'real-life' circumstances. Yet contemporary renditions of choice in childbirth frequently focus upon individual childbearing people, thereby reflecting and reiterating the intensely individualised responsibility of being a 'good mother' within contemporary capitalism. Rendered invisible in such iterations of choice are the structures, oppressions and reverberations (not to mention precarity and uncertainty) of a highly gendered, racial capitalism. Such dynamics also tend to be veiled when consideration is given to the topic of caesareans as requested by birthing people themselves.

'TOO POSH TO PUSH'?

Although many people end up giving birth by caesarean when they would have preferred not to, some people *do* want to have a caesarean section and plan for that with clinicians during their pregnancy. When a caesarean takes place at the request of the birthing parent in the absence of any apparent 'medical indication' (to use to terminology of the field), this is often referred to as a 'maternal request caesarean' or 'patient request caesarean'. Given that not all birthing people are mothers and the word 'patient' carries connotations of illness and passivity, neither terms are ideal. Nonetheless, the topic is important. When Birthrights, a UK-based organisation aimed at protecting human rights in pregnancy, conducted a survey in 2018, they found considerable variation in the ways in which hospitals were approaching this kind of caesarean, with some having a blanket policy of not accommodating maternal request caesareans.[52] As a result, there is considerable disparity in the extent to which people in different parts of the country could access this kind of caesarean: a veritable postcode lottery was seen to be operating, creating considerable anguish for a range of birthing people.

Over recent decades, people who decide to have a caesarean have been subject to various criticisms, including criticisms of the highly derogatory 'too posh to push' variety.[53] In a media analysis carried out in the UK between 1999 and 2011, it was found that various newspaper articles depicted maternal request caesareans (and sometimes wider elective caesareans for which there was a medical indication) as a 'lifestyle choice' – the suggestion being that birthing people were too busy or had 'too high powered a job to be able to allow the unpredictability of labor and birth to get in the way'.[54] If people are choosing caesareans for such reasons, that certainly speaks to the pressures and constraints of contemporary capitalism in various people's lives. Sociologist Katherine Beckett makes an important point when she argues that it is 'theoretically inadequate' to view people who opt for a caesarean as doing so because they have been socialised into 'dominant values'.[55] Women who would prefer to have an unmedicated vaginal birth are also accused of being socialised according to prevailing hegemonic values (e.g., of the 'natural birth' variety), and neither set of contentions is particularly helpful when it comes to actively supporting pregnant people. When gestational parents are asked *why* they request a caesarean, the reasons they give are far more nuanced than references to calendars, convenience and consumer culture even begin to suggest. Some consider themselves at high risk of having an emergency caesarean when in labour, and want to avoid that possibility.[56] Fear of birth looms large and not least as a result of traumatic events when previously giving birth.[57] References to poor care, inadequate communication and coercion by paid birth workers feature prominently in people's descriptions of traumatic birthing experiences.[58] Much birth trauma is iatrogenic (the product of service provision) and people request caesareans to avoid trauma of precisely that kind. In this respect, it may well be that people are planning to have abdominal births in very conscious and deliberate attempts to escape (understaffed) 'conveyor-belt care' or to avoid being treated simply as 'raw materials' in the production of babies. Planned abdominal birth does not entirely protect birthing people from being treated in such ways, but it does prevent a person from being subject to those possibilities whilst also in the throes of labour.

It merits mention in this context that when childbearing people are being treated in trauma-inducing ways, birth workers themselves may also be labouring in difficult conditions, be overworked and struggling with 'horizontal violence' as well as vertical power structures.[59] This is *not* an excuse.

The attitude and approach of individual birth workers makes an inordinate difference to the experiences of birthing people and their loved ones. Even on her deathbed, my grandmother recounted a painful memory of how a hospital matron had treated her after she gave birth. The event had taken place half a century earlier. It *is* worth emphasising however, that hospital hierarchies, staffing levels, workloads, the structuring of work processes and the social norms which prevail through particular maternity units, have a detrimental effect on birth workers as well as on pregnant people. A recent report instigated on maternity care failures at a particular NHS trust in England, identified many compounding issues including staff bullying, staff silencing and staff shortages.[60] So too has a 2024 report of the All-Party Parliamentary Group on Birth Trauma.[61] The conditions in which midwives and doctors labour are also those in which people birth and babies are born, and the injuries and suffering endured by gestational parents and their loved ones are intimately related to the working conditions of nurses, midwives, doctors, etc.[62] I'm not convinced that the language of 'choice' adequately enables such tangled relations to be considered.

'HOME ALONE'

When Tricia Anderson was reflecting upon childbearing choices over twenty years ago, she anticipated a situation in the not too distant future, in which many women feel they have little choice but to opt for a highly medicalised birth or to 'birth alone at home'.[63] She was concerned that those might be the only 'choices' left. It was a rhetorical point on which to end an article, and I am not suggesting that those are the only possibilities available to pregnant people today. Yet the underlying argument Anderson was making is important. While some people are today seeking to avoid labour 'care' by planning for a caesarean, others are avoiding the birthing services altogether for reasons that are decidedly similar. Statistics are not available on the scale and extent of what is now referred to as 'freebirthing' – intentionally birthing without midwives or doctors in attendance – but it is anticipated that rates are rising in parts of the Global North.[64] In some instances, freebirthing has been described as a 'positive choice' on the part of a childbearing person, but in many cases that terminology would be misleading.[65] If people feel they have no option but to freebirth because mainstream birth services are a site of trauma for them, or because services are not available which support their needs, it is debatable how much positive choice, or freedom for that matter, is involved. Yet as Anderson inquired all those years ago, if the babies of people birthing without health professionals struggle or die 'at whose door would you lay the blame?'[66] It was a pertinent question to pose. There is widespread stigmatisation of people who birth outside of formal healthcare systems, and that is the case even when babies are born entirely healthy. In England, freebirth is legal, but that does not prevent people being reported to social services on child protection grounds when they deliberately birth without doctors or midwives in attendance.[67]

Whatever systemic problems plague healthcare systems and hospitals, few pregnant people – if any – would choose to have their access to those services actively hindered if they needed, or wanted, to use such facilities. Yet in England, many migrant groups are unable to receive care through the National Health Service without being burdened with hefty debts that they simply cannot pay.[68] In Aotearoa New Zealand, people are often required to make payments towards even many clinically indicated pregnancy ultrasound scans, contributing to inequitable access to those provisions.[69] In the US, there are considerable out-of-pocket expenses for perinatal services, even for people who have health insurance coverage (and not all do). The medical debt accrued by people as a result of perinatal care bills, is a significant problem – and particularly, it would seem, for those who are on low incomes and/or who have specific health conditions that are closely associated with poverty.[70] However celebrated 'choice' may be in contemporary capitalism, there are substantial constraints on the choices of many pregnant people.

STATE COERCION

Some 'choices' are also the subject of long legal battles or are quite simply illegal, and this has been notoriously so in the US: the land, apparently, of the free. Even prior to the overturning of *Roe v. Wade* (which eliminated the federal constitutional right to abortion) so-called 'fetal protection laws' have been operating at state level. Generally speaking, where such laws are in place, a person can be prosecuted if something they did whilst pregnant is deemed to have caused harm to the foetus. Under legislation of this kind, people have been arrested and/or prosecuted for acts as diverse as declining to have a caesarean section or for taking drugs during pregnancy, *even if such actions cannot be shown to have caused harm to the foetus*.[71] Between 1973 and 2005, the vast majority of US cases in which a person was arrested or subject to forced medical interventions (including caesarean) on grounds such as these, were levelled against poor working-class women; of those cases in which data pertaining to race were available, nearly 60 per cent of cases were against Women of Colour and more specifically 52 per cent were against African-American women.[72] Well over half of the cases were instigated in the southern states of the US. In the words of law professor Michele Goodwin, 'where planters once controlled Black women's reproduction on their plantations and elsewhere, now the state controls what Black women (and others) may do with their bodies during pregnancy.'[73] In the context of a highly racial capitalism, choice is far from celebrated for all.

The idea that legislation and actions of the so-called 'fetal protection' variety actually support the health of a foetus is ill-founded. If support around drug use in pregnancy is not available, or if pregnant people are reluctant to access prenatal care for fear of being accused of causing foetal harm, the health of future generations is hardly being taken seriously. In the words of researchers who have studied the effects of Tennessee's 2014 so-called Fetal Assault Law: 'We find consistent evidence that this law undermined the ability of mothers to access prenatal care, worsened birth outcomes, and increased both fetal and infant death rates.'[74] I'm not alone in considering there to be far more effective ways of supporting future generations than threatening, coercing, punishing and imprisoning their gestational parents. As Goodwin enquires in the US, 'how are shackling, birthing in prison toilets, and rearing children behind bars demonstrative of the state's respect or care for fetal or child life?'[75] Such events and practices are not demonstrative of respect for the health of childbearing people either.

The criminalisation of abortion has widespread implications for incarcerated peoples as well as for childbirth beyond prison walls. Since Roe v. Wade was overturned by the US Supreme Court in 2022, the access imprisoned people have to abortion has become even more precarious and restricted than was previously the case.[76] Outside of prisons, lack of abortion access also has profound health effects. If abortion is not available, far more unwanted pregnancies continue to term than previously the case and many of these will be the pregnancies of people for whom quality health and pregnancy care, as well as abortion, is limited. Even prior to 2022, maternal and infant death rates were higher in states with the most restrictive abortion legislation and disproportionately impacted Women of Colour in comparison to white women.[77] There is significant concern amongst US obstetricians that the 2022 Supreme Court ruling has made it more difficult for them to deal with obstetric emergencies, has negatively impacted upon maternal mortality and has exacerbated already existing racial inequities in pregnancy-related contexts.[78] In many US states at the time of writing, even when a pregnancy involves a life- or health-threatening complication, abortions are inaccessible or difficult to obtain.[79] Perhaps it is unsurprising that safe abortion is now referred to as a basic human right, however difficult that right is to attain in various parts of the world. In so far as childbirth and abortion are concerned, the language of 'choice' fails to indicate the gravity of the issues at stake.

COORDINATES OF CHOICE

As the forces of capitalist production developed and a vast range of commodities and knowledge forms proliferated, discourses celebrating individual choice became integral to the ideological infrastructure of an increasingly neoliberal capitalism. Within that environment, certain choices became heavily normalised, expected even (at least for certain social groups), whilst others were stigmatised and difficult to realise or attain. Within hierarchically premised health services where 'assembly line' structures shape the work processes of many health professionals, choice merged painfully with coercion in many birthing places. Choices have never been equally available for all. If white, wealthy women are structurally privileged in so far as choice in childbirth is concerned, so too are many able-bodied women. Research demonstrates that conditions which support people to determine key aspects of their own birthing process are less accessible for disabled people than they are for many non-disabled pregnant people.[80] Yet as advocates of social models of disability have argued for decades now, relations and environments supporting self-determination are precisely what is required to *prevent* a social context from being actively disabling.

Prevailing heteronormative assumptions also restrict the choices that are available to many people within the perinatal services. Despite pregnancy and birthing services often being referred to as '*maternity* services', the institutional structure of these services seldom accommodates the reality that a baby may have *two* mothers or that a non-birthing person may be the *mother* of an infant.[81] By a similar token, the experiences of transgender and non-binary people who are pregnant are frequently rendered invisible within those services and there are blatant examples of transphobia within such spaces.[82] A key way in which trans and non-binary people act to keep themselves safe when navigating the perinatal services, is by deliberately searching for and choosing a primary care provider with a community reputation for practicing in ways which are affirming and inclusive. Some speak of deciding to birth at home supported by a midwife with whom they have built a trusting relationship, thereby minimising contact with the wider service context.[83] That may not be possible in countries or areas where there are no midwives or where midwives are actively constrained or prevented from attending births at home. Aspects of pregnancy and childbearing can, but don't always, heighten gender dysphoria, and some trans men decide to have an elective (pre-labour) caesarean as a way of determining their own birthing process.[84] Whatever choices are made, not having access to supportive perinatal care is quite simply unsafe. At the same time, restricted access to and very legitimate fear of unsafe care, shapes the 'choices' that many people make and are able to make around childbirth.

A UK survey conducted during the COVID-19 pandemic, with parents who were either expecting or had just had a baby, found that participants within the LGBTQ+ community were more likely than cisheterosexual respondents to actively consider freebirthing.[85] As the coronavirus spread across the world, obstetric hospitals changed (and restricted) their policies around the presence of birthing partners, birthing unit staffing levels were impacted by illness, home-birth services were halted and hospitals were also sites where the virus prevailed. Such factors contributed to freebirthing being considered by a range of people who had not previously contemplated that possibility. In this context, LGBTQ+ persons were left to face the cisheteronormativity of birth institutions without the trusted support and advocacy they had planned for, thereby creating additional inequities. Moreover, the COVID regulations did not account for the necessities of diverse family structures. One survey respondent voiced concerns that may have been relevant to many: as a lactating parent who was not gestating, would she be permitted access to the hospital to feed the newborn baby?[86] The pandemic exacerbated a range of structural constraints and lack of 'choice' that were already operative in relation to childbearing anyway.

CONTRADICTIONS OF CAPITALISM, CATASTROPHE AND CHOICE

The COVID-19 pandemic is not the only apparently 'natural' disaster of epic proportions to have impacted birthing people, and the population more generally, over recent years. Events such as large-scale flooding and intense tropical cyclones have become increasingly commonplace across the world, affecting the extent to which people can access birth services in different parts of the globe. In crisis-ridden regions, including those devastated by war or earthquakes, as well as by extreme weather events, people often birth their babies before they reach hospital or before birth workers arrive to support them, and the possibilities of birthing in hospital can be severely disrupted by such realities as power outages, generator failures, supply-chain blockages and resource shortages. When Cyclone Gabrielle devastated areas of Aotearoa New Zealand in 2023, people who had planned to have their babies in hospitals or birth centres gave birth at home instead, as others made their way or were airlifted to birthing units in treacherous conditions; some birth workers could not arrive at their place of employment, whilst others could not leave.[87] Of course, the babies kept on coming. Births may seldom make headline news in disaster situations, yet childbirth continues to happen even when the contours of people's lives are disrupted into chaos and lie in ruin.[88] It may be stating the obvious to note that in conditions such as these a person's choices around birth are heavily curtailed, and the point I want to emphasise extends beyond that. In short, capitalism is *actively producing* crises which explode and annihilate the very choices and possibilities around parturition that have been generated *by* that mode of production in the first place.

In addition to the decimations of war and genocide, the realities of environmental collapse currently and urgently beckon the end of capitalism as a globalised totality and therefore the annihilation of so many of the birthing 'choices' produced (at least for some) by this economic system. Capitalism is a mode of production premised upon the violent and ongoing severing of people from the land, the relentless pursuit of profit and economic growth through exploited labour combined with technologies that (so often) depend upon fossil fuel, and in which the dumping of waste production materials in rivers, seas and across lands has been heavily normalised. Whilst various commentators emphasise *human activity* as causal of contemporary environmental crisis, I'm not alone in finding such arguments problematic.[89] Human beings have lived on the planet for millennia without altering the course of geologic history and without creating the levels of environmental devastation currently contended with. At the present time, people in the Global South contribute far less greenhouse gas emissions than do those in the Global North (whilst disproportionately experiencing the effects of rising sea levels and of environmental breakdown more generally). Placing responsibility for climate change upon the activity of generic human beings (as if humans and their activity were entirely uniform and undifferentiated) renders invisible the extent to which people's actions are shaped and determined by political-economic context, and the degree to which people today do not equally contribute to global warming. However repetitious such an argument may be, people's activities *are* powerfully informed by the gendered, racial and imperialist configurations of contemporary capitalism, and it would be a complicit erasure of the power of capital and an overlooking of inequitable resource distribution to ignore that. So it is that while I wholeheartedly support the (often political) decision of people who do not want to bear children for environmental reasons, I also consider it deeply problematic for such a course of action to be imposed on all. In this I am reminded of the anti-Malthusian arguments against a birth-strike. Individual decision-making – choice even – is important when it comes to childbearing, but capitalism rather than population (or a universalising account of human activity) is the crux of so many of the issues which currently plague planet and people alike.

The role of capital in climate change is brought into sharp focus when specific contradictions are emphasised. For instance, I find it useful to be reminded of the current time as one in which humans have become so apparently powerful as to have decidedly altered the environmental course of the planet, whilst also appearing *incapable* of acting together in ways which will halt or reverse the damage caused.[90] Despite large bodies of science and knowledge regarding what needs to be done to tackle climate change, entire countries are systematically failing to cut their greenhouse gas emissions in anywhere near the quantities required.[91] This is more than an ironic twist of fate. We live in an era in which powerful capitalists are responsible for vast amounts of carbon emissions through their investments in fossil-fuel and related industries.[92] It is one thing to place responsibility with consumers to live and purchase more ethically, and quite another to hold capitalists themselves to account, to ensure the availability and affordability of sustainable products, and to restructure work and land distribution in such ways as people have time, skills and resources to build their lives in ways which support and enhance the ecosystems to which they are integral. At the current time, it would certainly seem that capital's relentless drive to accumulate – the prioritisation of short-term motivations of profit over planet – holds more sway and influence than do collectively reasoned plans for climate action, and I'm not entirely convinced that Marx would have considered that strange. He understood that whilst people do not make history exactly as they please, under capitalism humans also become estranged from the very characteristics which define their species: from their capacity to act together in conscious and deliberately planned ways *with* the object of the entire species, and other species, in mind. The point to be emphasised in this context is not that capitalist states are failing to hold billionaire polluters to account, although that is so. Marx indicated that within capitalism people become alienated from their very *species being.* Today, many people have very little option but to sell their capacity for conscious human activity (in the form of their ability to work), so that they and their immediate kin can survive. In that respect, people's conscious life activity comes to be focused on work for employers – on work that so often produces capital – rather than on work for the collective long-term well-being of people and the planet. Capital also has vampire-like tendencies: sucking from and shaping the activities of those who created it. This is not to say that people are entirely impotent in the face of capital, but rather to acknowledge that capital does have considerable influence over the ways in which people live their lives, birth and *choose* today.

As much as capital is plagued with contradiction, so too is childbirth within social formations where capital predominates. Humans have always acted with conscious deliberation in relation to childbirth, but it was in the context of late twentieth-century capitalism that a range of social circumstances amalgamated in such ways as choice in childbirth came to be lauded, extolled and celebrated around parturition. Capitalism provided conditions through which a range of childbearing choices became apparently possible, even if they were not necessarily entirely desirable (or obtainable). Moreover, capitalism is now producing crises in which such choices may be eliminated anyway. In this, I am reminded of the remarkable capacity of the capitalist mode of production to disturb and transform even the conditions of its own existence. When it comes to the drive, dynamism and destructive capabilities of this political-economic system, nothing – it would seem – is sacred: 'All that is solid melts into air, all that is holy is profaned … .'[93] Perhaps it is unsurprising therefore, that scholars and birth workers are currently inquiring as to what happens in childbirth when all that has been built-up and reified over recent decades, when all that has been produced and deemed necessary, is no longer tenable:

> When the clock on the wall that indicated time for another cervical check lies shattered and the electricity for monitoring mother and fetus is down, what tools will sustain us? When epidemics and pandemics add to the preexisting risks of hospitals as sites of contagion, where indeed should the mothers give birth?[94]

These researchers indicate that childbirth in disaster situations – the kinds of situations which are increasingly normalised within contemporary capitalism – frequently require responses of the low-tech, highly socialised variety.

Which is to say that disaster environments call for highly committed and skilled care (particularly midwifery) across a range of locations, the facilitation of arrangements so people can access sites of obstetric care if necessary, and large amounts of adaptability on the part of childbearing people, their families, local communities and all involved. In this respect, the importance of 'low-tech, high-touch' care is emphasised.[95] Such care may well involve corporeal touch, but touch in this context also means establishing and maintaining relationships and networks of communication involving birthing people, their families, loved ones, birth workers, local support organisations, disaster relief operations, etc. Technologies will be used, but technological fetishism is largely redundant in circumstances such as these. As writers on global childbearing health are now emphasising:

> Providing 'high touch' health care to women and infants does not mean eschewing technology, but it does mean not allowing technology to drive the intervention. It also means resisting the temptation to think that more and better technologies can substitute for a commitment to high touch.[96]

They note that despite the benefits of RCTs in various service contexts, rigid adherence to RCT findings falls considerably short of supporting understanding of viable possibilities across terrains that are remarkably different from one another. Despite the tendency in capitalism for the intensely social relations which connect people to be rendered opaque and invisible (which is precisely the premise of Marxist readings of fetish), capitalism is now *actively generating* crises and catastrophes in which relations and connections between people *must* be highlighted, prioritised and brought to the foreground as a matter of safety. Emphasis upon risk, evidence and, of course, choice also assume radically different contours in situations such as these. Disaster contexts, and their normalisation, shed new light on 'what is to be done' when it comes to childbirth within, and beyond, the parameters of the currently prevalent mode of production.

7
From the 'Womb' of the Present ...

A new society is not delivered by the stork. The beginnings – the precursors and antecedents – of what is to come, grow in the world that is already with us. Futures gestate in the present as much as we move and act to create change in conditions given and inherited. It was once famously noted that new social relations of production become possible once 'the material conditions of their existence have matured in the womb of the old society.'[1] Let's hope they mature soon: given the urgencies imposed by climate change, they might need a bit of a push. Immanent necessity now calls on people to work deliberately and consciously together: to act collectively to encourage and usher in futures without the violence, appropriation and exploitation of today. But given how intensely social the birthing of individual people – as well as of societies – can be, gestational imagery of the kind deployed by Marx can also be turned around. If the social relations of the future gestate in the 'womb' of the current society, the intensely social relations of the present *also* make their presence felt upon and through the bodies of actual childbearing people. Networks of relationships that are largely unseen, shape the conditions in which people birth; they influence the ways in which a person's childbearing body and self might stretch, tear, be cut, or heal. They meld with the twists and turns of a new person's arrival into the extra-uterine world. However unseen such relations and determinations might be, they inform the ways in which new mothers, parents and people are birthed and thrive into the future – or not. Those tractions and relationships are far from static; they alter across time and space, and will yet be subject to change – disruption even. Given this, birthing is more than a metaphor for social change. Birthing is also a site of very tangible political struggle and for social transformation.

No single chapter, text or tome, could highlight all of the groups, social movements and projects involved in activism around childbirth today. To draw this book to a close, I draw attention to just a few: to some of the ways in which childbearing people, birth workers and their supporters have been and continue to be collectively energised to improve the conditions in which people grow babies, birth, labour and live. Marxists have often prioritised so-called 'productive activity', as performed in factories, in their formulations of post-capitalist societies, but childbearing people and birth workers also have skills and knowledge crucial for the creation of futures in which exploitation and oppression are refused. Prior to developing this argument further, I begin by re-sketching and drawing together some of the considerations and deliberations developed in preceding chapters ... .

HISTORY HURTS

As forces of production have surged in and through capitalist landscapes, so too has the sheer volume of tools, technologies and products available on markets and in obstetric spaces. Some of these commodities are crucial – at times – in mediating childbirth to support the well-being of people, but lurking beneath their production, sale, purchase and deployment are powerful forces unrelated to the optimisation of health: pressures to maximise capital accumulation, to boost health-worker productivity, to deal with short-staffing in obstetric units already structured to maximise 'patient throughput', and to soothe the fears (even line the pockets) of health professionals. Irish author and travel writer Dervla Murphy contends that the financial interests and relationships embroiled in 'the birth industry' are more complex still than those which sustain the tobacco industry: 'Think Big Pharma ... plus certain subterranean relationships between *some* of the obstetric fraternity and *some* multinational purveyors of medical equipment and *some* representatives of the insurance industry.'[2] She is not wrong. Structurally related to such vested interests are also dynamics of profound neglect. Capitalism has spread across the globe imposing iatrogenic excess where profit might be made, whilst many birthing people are denied access to even the basics of safe healthcare.

As medical technologies have been generated for the accumulation of capital, they have also been produced for the identification, management and proliferation of risk. That is, risk which operates – so often – as a proximate indication of structural inequality, neglect, misogyny and racism through the lives and bodies of childbearing people. As risk surges through the financial calculations of corporate and state-related entities (of insurance companies, hospital administrations, etc.), products – more and more of them – are purchased and deployed across the terrain of perinatal services. These are 'risk-management' tools, as well as commodified and commercially articulated responses to generations of socially exacerbated and economically created problems. In best-case scenarios, scientific evidence supports and validates the usage and deployment of these tools. But beware of guidelines and hospital protocols that are *not* based upon evidence, and of evidence informed by the profit drive of pharmaceutical or medical tech companies. As neoliberal capitalism gathered momentum, no wonder people campaigned and rallied for women to have *choice* in how they birth. Twentieth-century capitalism was drawing to a close; the burgeoning of data and knowledge extraction technologies had enhanced public accessibility to health information; and calls for women to *choose* what was done to their labouring bodies was a largely progressive articulation of the times. Yet choice also liaised with consumerist logic, and calls for individuals to choose the conditions of their labours did not challenge – as some had hoped they might – the deeply structural relations which constrain birthing in contemporary capitalism, nor which generate vast gestational inequities. As capitalism encounters contradictions of its own creating, some of the choices that some people were able to make are now being eradicated anyway.

'History is what hurts', wrote Fredric Jameson in 1981.[3] I do not quote his words in order to deny that childbirth hurts, but to emphasise that human childbirth *is* history. As people birth, their labours are shaped and morphed by social forces and relations that can be incredibly painful – even deadly. Black women do not die at higher rates in childbearing than white women because of anything 'natural' about bodies and birth, but because of the violence of racism – of racial colonial capitalism – surging through living and birthing spaces. Individualised blame still prevails when pregnancy or birth 'goes wrong': it is far less socially and systemically disruptive to pour scorn on individual people – and not least on Women of Colour – than to challenge the profoundly inequitable relations of a racialised, gendered and disabling capitalism. Perhaps it is for reasons such as this that many birth workers consider their attendance at births to be, in itself, a form of activism. That is, activism with aspiration and resolve to hold at bay many of the social forces that have been discussed in this book: pressures of understaffing, protocols unfounded on evidence, torrents of risk, systemic racism, homophobia, transphobia … the list continues. All of these dynamics and more may be eddying and heaving outside of a birth room. But sometimes, just sometimes, the door can be closed (at times very literally) and the detrimental effects of those powerful influences on a birthing person can be blocked and minimised. This is the kind of work sometimes described as 'holding space'. It is the labour of safeguarding a birthing environment – be that a house, a room, or an emotional milieu – so that people can do the work of birthing a baby in ways that they, as far as is ever possible, determine for themselves. Silvia Federici makes a related point in contending that:

> ... birth work is above all a transformative, autonomy-building activity, enabling women to 'take charge of their reproductive journey,' overcome their fears, discover their inner powers, turn the moment in which they are most vulnerable into one in which they can be strongest and, thereby begin a process of self-valorization.[4]

I do not underestimate the powerful effects that a birth in which a child-bearing person feels strong, powerful and flourishing can have upon the health and well-being of that person, and of those they love. Yet I am not sure people are ever *entirely* autonomous of social and economic forces, nor of their bodies, as they gestate corporeally and socially within any society. There is an intensely political, as well as strategic, need to defend principles of self-determination in birthing spaces. But if History hurts, that is precisely because History constrains the parameters of possibility – 'sets inexorable limits to individual as well as collective praxis'.[5] Given such dynamics and their effects on parturition, many birth workers also understand that their activism does not end when they leave a birth and that it must not focus exclusively on pregnant people. As well as attending births, birth workers are also involved in ongoing struggles to prevent the closure of local hospitals and community birthing facilities. In some parts of the world, midwives are campaigning and lobbying for insurance coverage so they can work at all; they are resisting the criminalisation of birth workers – including the incarceration of those who support people to birth at home, outside of mainstream hospital services. The contemporary activism of birth workers extends well beyond that which immediately supports people as they gestate, birth and care for new generations. Some of that activist work, as well as constraints thereby encountered, are sketched in the discussion that follows ... .

WHAT IS BEING DONE?

Over the past decade nurses, midwives and doctors have taken strike action across a range of countries. In doing so, they have rallied against a cascade of pressures which limit the parameters of their work: below-inflation pay offers, lack of pay equity, understaffed working conditions, etc. They have challenged capitalist priorities which impact upon public-sector institutions, as state support for even basic health services has been eroded and delegitimised. Birth workers do not strike simply for pay rises or better hours (although both can be incredibly important), but to protect childbearing people, their loved ones and public safety generally. Strike action is a way of pushing back against conditions in which staff have 'no time to care': no time to work with pregnant people in ways that are safe, supportive and nourishing for all involved.[6] In short, birth workers strike *because* they care.[7] Yet not all birth workers are employees – some work as solo practitioners or in group practices, and have no employer against whom to take industrial action. If the labour processes of many paid birth workers are structured akin to factory production processes, neither do improved staffing levels and better remuneration resolve the problems of childbearing people. Other forms of activism are also required to transform the spaces of parturition.

Many birth workers and birth activists are seeking to end the coercion that childbearing people are subject to as they birth. In Latin America, movements have been successful in developing laws which specifically legislate against *obstetric violence.*[8] Obstetric violence is variously defined but broadly pertains to abusive (some prefer to use the word 'disrespectful') behaviour – including forced treatments, shouting, swearing and hitting – to which birthing people are subject within the 'maternity services'. Even in countries where obstetric violence is not named in law, these forms of 'treatment' are a violation of human rights. In the terms of international law and by contemporary legal standards, many of the issues raised in this book (such as preventable deaths, forced interventions, systemic neglect of birthing people and many of the effects of 'conveyor-belt care') are flagrant violations of human rights. A range of human rights birth-related court cases have now been won across different countries: cases pertaining to maternal death, to how and where people birth, and to pay equity for midwives.[9] Notwithstanding the importance of these wins, legal approaches to birth equity, safety and justice harbour a range of limitations. Many childbearing people do not have the means to wage legal battles against states or service providers. Legal activism has a crucial role to play, but it is one thing for rights to be declared and emboldened by statutes, and it is quite another for the social conditions to be achieved in which those rights are realised for all.

In the 1980s and 1990s, birth activists in Aotearoa New Zealand adopted a rather different approach to improving birth care. Rather than appealing to human rights, they sought to radically restructure the maternity services.[10] A unique model of publicly funded care was thereby established. Instead of people being pushed along a conveyor-belt system – being seen by scores of health professionals and birthing in a hospital staffed by complete strangers – the maternity services were structured so that childbearing people could decide *who* they wanted to be their primary birth worker and that health worker would walk with them, so to speak, on their childbearing journey. The 'Lead Maternity Carer' (LMC) meets with the childbearing person regularly throughout their pregnancy and for weeks afterwards, may well be present at the birth, and coordinates with other specialists involved in providing care.[11] Most people have a midwife as their LMC, and words such as 'partnership' and 'reciprocity' have been readily used to describe the relationship of pregnant women and their midwife.[12] Yet Aotearoa New Zealand has not been immune to the pressures which contemporary capitalism exerts on perinatal services globally and there are serious midwifery workforce deficits across the land.[13] Activity is ongoing to address midwife shortages, and in particular to increase numbers of Māori and Pasifika midwives, so that they are equitably represented within the workforce.[14] Work also continues to ensure and develop cultural safety across the health services – that is, care which meets the self-defined needs of tangata whenua (Māori) and, following from that, of all people.[15] Culturally safe care is decidedly not conveyor-belt care. In the words of Irihapeti Ramsden, the nurse who developed the notion of cultural safety, cultural safety pertains to 'life chances' rather than 'lifestyles'; integral to that is 'access to health services, education and decent housing within an environment in which it is safe to be born brown'.[16] In the context of perinatal care, a key aspect of cultural safety involves ensuring that whānau (a childbearing person *in the context of* their own extended family and/or self-defined networks of support people), rather than women individualised and severed from the relations that most nurture them, are incorporated into the processes of care. I am not convinced that everybody in Aotearoa New Zealand understands how important and profound the very premises of cultural safety are.

In the US, the birthing justice movement has developed as part of the reproductive justice movement.[17] Activists speak of the birth justice movement as 'rooted in black and brown communities' and as forging 'a new vision of reproductive freedom'.[18] That vision is 'of a decolonized people, shaking off colonial and patriarchal legacies, challenging racial inequities, and building new relationships defined not by commerce but by commitments to social justice, community empowerment, and love as an insurgent praxis'.[19] Integral to the tenets of birthing justice is the premise that pregnant people are able to determine whether they continue with their pregnancy, and – if they do – how and with whom they give birth. Birth justice groups are seeking to improve access to midwives and doulas within their own communities: 'Community-based doula care reflects an organized, collective framework where African American, African immigrant/refugee, Latinx, Indigenous or historically underserved individuals formalize and implement programs with the specific aim of serving their own communities.'[20] Not all doulas work from such radical premises. Community doulas are integral to the communities they serve and they understand well how poverty, racism, housing, incarceration and immigration shape people's lives and health around birth and beyond. They support people in their homes, transform medical jargon into accessible information, ascertain whether families have enough to eat, and link them with broader networks and organisations of support.[21] They stand by people as they enter the hospital system, seeking to ensure their voices are heard and their needs met amidst the clamouring of risk algorithms, the depersonalisation of productivity drives, technocratic responses to deeply social problems and ongoing systemic racism. Projects now support doulas to work in prisons, and some have established doula mentorship and training for people who have previously been imprisoned.[22]

Doulas are a key component of contemporary strategies for tackling birth inequities, but it is difficult to maintain economic viability as a doula working exclusively in low-income communities.[23] In precisely the areas where doulas are most needed, many people cannot afford to pay for their services at rates which ensure the work is sustainable.[24] Calls for Medicaid to cover doula services are ongoing, yet even when such coverage is achieved, reimbursements rates are not always sufficient for doulas to earn a living wage.[25] Many doulas report feeling 'unwelcome and disrespected while practicing in hospital settings'.[26] As one explains, 'My biggest obstacle is if I'm in the labor room, if I'm really an advocate [laughs], I'll get thrown out.'[27] Doulas also do much of the work that other birth workers, *if they had the time*, would love to do. For some nurses, a doula being present in a birthing room is said to signal 'further loss of contact with their patients, in an environment [already] dominated by technology and diminished patient interaction'.[28] Yet doulas are not responsible for the array of social forces and relations that coalesce in busy obstetric hospitals. Moreover, despite pressures upon doula communities to improve perinatal outcomes, the work of resolving crises which have been systemically generated over decades is beyond the capacity of any individual person or single group of workers to achieve.[29] Many midwives, nurses and doctors *do* advocate for doulas, while also highlighting the necessity of wider transformations in the conditions and configurations of contemporary pregnancy and birth care, such as increases in the funding and measures available to support community-based midwifery. The vast majority of people need more care and support in this era of relentless extraction, accumulation and crisis.

It may also be that doulas, particularly in some parts of the world and particularly those working primarily in non-hospital locations, are currently doing the work of maintaining and preserving skills and knowledge that may have previously been considered the domain of midwifery. That is to say, the kinds of skills that are increasingly difficult for midwives to perform in understaffed hospitals – but that are much needed if non-violent, safe birthing for all, is to be a possibility. As one UK-based doula explains:

> ... when I started this, I saw myself as a doula that could fill a gap, that doulas were a stopgap until they got maternity services sorted out. And now in some ways I feel like doulas are the last threads of midwifery. Kind of holding on to some of the knowledge. Some of the wisdom. Some of the tools that midwifery is no longer allowed to use or they don't have time to use. Like sitting patiently, like knitting, like not asking questions and just being there.[30]

The pressures of contemporary capitalism certainly make it very difficult for many midwives to do the work of being calmly present through somebody's labour and waiting for birthing to unfurl. Yet, as an experienced and well-respected midwife shared with me, one of the most difficult and crucial skills she learned in attending births was how to sit on her hands. That is hardly the labour that generates value for capital – and it is work largely unappreciated in busy obstetric units. But it is integral to 'holding space', and in so far as the health of childbearing people and babies are concerned, it may well be safer and far more effective – *if done strategically and at appropriate times* – than many of the tasks currently prioritised in the prevailing spaces of parturition. If the nurturing of traditional midwifery skills continue to be unprioritised within the mainstream UK health services, it seems quite likely that current trends in the direction of freebirthing will continue. It must *not* be assumed that only white middle-class women will (or do) move into the freebirthing space.

In the UK, struggles are ongoing to save the National Health Service, and importantly so. If the publicly owned health system were to be further transferred into the hands of profit-seeking capitalists, many of the problems which currently haunt the 'maternity services' would be further exacerbated. The NHS was the 'national treasure' of the post-Second World War period

– that is, an era in which the state invested substantially in the (re)production of a healthy workforce. It was never perfect but in so far as healthcare in capitalism goes, the principles of the NHS – funded by general taxation and 'free at the point of use' – are hard to beat and well worth defending. The era in which the capitalist state sought to actively 'look after' the national workforce have long since passed, and decades of financialisation, and neoliberal and austerity politics have left the National Health Service in a painful state of disrepair. In 2023, 87 per cent of the 3,949 midwives and maternity service workers who responded to a survey on working conditions, reported that staffing levels in their workplace were *not safe*.[31] That is a huge proportion. It is far easier to convince the public that privatisation is the best course of action, when a public service has already been broken. Midwives and their supporters took to the streets in 2022, calling on the government to invest in, and implement a range of measures to support, the perinatal services. As one doula involved in organising the demonstration noted, there are high rates of trauma amongst birthing people and nervous breakdowns amongst maternity service staff. She pertinently added: 'midwives' working conditions are families' birthing conditions.'[32] It is a maxim that cannot be repeated enough.

In acknowledgement of some of the pressures to which health workers are currently subjected, trade union work is ongoing to address the bullying and harassment of health workers within the workplace. There is also activist work supporting midwives subject to disciplinary investigations by their employer or regulatory authority.[33] Those involved in this form of activism suggest that some midwives may be more likely to have their practice investigated than others *not* because of incompetence, but because these midwives resist 'the ever-increasing impetus to process women' through the maternity system: that is to say, *process* rather than support women to birth in ways that are right for *them*.[34] In creating a safe haven for midwives under scrutiny, powerful connections are being acknowledged between the mechanisms via which midwives are controlled and regulated in the workplace, and the coercion endured by many childbearing people as they themselves encounter, or are 'processed through' (perhaps not unlike raw materials), these service contexts.

Birth workers are also involved in supporting their colleagues and childbearing people who are working, labouring and trying to survive against forces of imperialism and colonialism, particularly in war zones, across the world. For instance, when Russia invaded Ukraine in 2022, Ukrainian midwives were not licensed to attend home-births, and as a result many lacked the experience and skills to support people to birth safely outside of hospitals – in their basements or air-raid shelters, for example.[35] Yet as health facilities were bombed and infrastructure devastated, that was precisely the kind of support that many pregnant women most needed. Ukrainian midwives have been working with Polish birth workers and others, to develop home-birth knowledge and skills, including skills in attending vaginal breech birthing.[36] As I write the final pages of this book, a range of pregnancy and birth workers are standing in solidarity with the people of Palestine as Israel continues its attacks on Gaza.[37] In February 2024, at least 28,340 Palestinians had been killed in Gaza over the previous four months, and it was reported that 70 per cent of them were women and children.[38] By the end of May, the death toll in Gaza had risen to 36,224 and huge numbers continue to be women and children.[39] The violence did not begin on 7 October 2023, when Hamas carried out its cross-border attack. As a US-based reproductive care organisation has noted, reproductive justice involves people having 'the right to parent their children in safe and healthy environments, free from oppression, exploitation, and state violence – the settler-colonial occupation makes this impossible.'[40] Even before the end of 2023 in Gaza, repeated attacks by the Israeli military had led to many health facilities being forced to close or operate without power, caesareans were being conducted without anaesthesia, and large numbers of Palestinian women were birthing without access to emergency facilities.[41] Rates of medical complications – such as pre-term birth and very low birthweight in babies – have escalated since, not least because women are malnourished in pregnancy and living in unfathomably stressful conditions.[42] At the same time as medical and emergency facilities are most needed by childbearing people and babies, they are least available – hospitals destroyed, lying in ruins with medical and fuel supplies blocked. Now, more than ever, resistance must be fertile.[43]

In addition to working in war zones, midwives are first responders when so-called 'natural' disasters strike across the world and some are also actively campaigning against climate change.[44] In so doing, they are working in conjunction with hospitals to reduce facility carbon emissions and calling for fossil fuel divestment. The very work of midwifery has a relatively low carbon footprint, not least because midwives often provide relatively low-tech, community-based care thereby minimising transport and carbon emissions. A well-supported midwifery workforce can also facilitate the creation of health and well-being (rather than simply the mitigation of risk), and help to build and nurture the strength and power of pregnant people, their loved ones and communities as they make birthing safe in ways that matter *for them.*

Such birthing looks very different from services which structurally protect the profits of med-tech companies and of corporations directly investing in fossil fuels.

BIRTHING NEW RELATIONS

As many examples of birth activism demonstrate, birth workers are often deeply committed to acting in ways which challenge the status quo. Integral to this, many have values and aspirations that are difficult to realise and nurture within the confines of contemporary capitalism. Developments towards increased perinatal equity or better birthing do not require the complete overthrow of capitalism, but capitalism *does* place limitations upon what it is possible to achieve within the current mode of production. A range of undertakings, strategies and structures are feasible within capitalism provided, as David Harvey notes, '*that they do not unduly restrict or destroy the capacity to produce surplus-value on an ever-expanding scale*.'[45] The italics are his. Capitalism's dependence on the continual expansion of surplus-value raises questions, for example, about how far it will be possible, within this mode of production, to entirely eradicate such injustices as 'too little, too late and too much, too soon'.[46] How far is that feasible if the capitalist expansion of surplus-value simultaneously involves the production of extreme wealth, excess and coercion, as well as poverty and neglect? Given structural dynamics such as these, there is potentially much to be gained from tracing and developing connections and overlaps between the work of people who attend births regularly and the work of activists who are exploring non-capitalist alternatives or who are explicitly challenging capitalism. The process of drawing and making such connections is already happening. For instance, the Critical Midwifery Collective Writing Group recently put out a call for papers for an upcoming edition of a major birth journal:

> We call on midwives, and other midwifery practitioners, scholars, and theorists to join our effort to achieve just and equitable SRMN [sexual, reproductive, maternal and newborn] care by developing Critical Midwifery Studies as an explicit field of academic inquiry and emancipatory praxis.[47]

Critical midwifery studies, they indicate, includes anti-racist, postcolonial as well as anti-capitalist critique. As an overlapping group of birth workers, scholars and activists also explain: 'We write in transnational solidarity with one another, aware of the impact of the capitalist, racist, and misogynist global reality that reproduces itself through institutions like obstetrics.'[48]

Yet much of the work of birth workers and activists is not written on paper or screens. For that reason alone, there will be far more overlaps and collaborations between birth activists and people seeking to challenge capitalism than it is possible to glean from literature or internet searches. I often find myself wondering about the interconnections that might already exist between, on the one hand, birth workers and on the other hand, people striving to keep the wealth they produce *within* their own communities – through such ventures, for example, as local cooperatives, enterprises democratically run by workers and networks of such initiatives.[49] Structures of this kind support workers and communities to determine *how* they produce goods and wealth, and how the products of that labour are distributed. Through such ventures – often referred to as the creation of solidarity economies – emphasis is upon people determining the conditions in which they make *products*. In locally based midwifery, emphasis is upon people determining the conditions in which they make *people*. I often think about the powerful combinations that might be possible if both were brought together. Perhaps they already are.

Marxists have often viewed factory employees as primary agents of anti-capitalist struggle – and they are crucial. But capital accumulation relies upon vast numbers of workers who are based in homes, hospitals and non-factory environments, and many whose work is not paid at all. When people working in non-factory environments down tools, they can also hold governments as well as capital to account in powerful ways. If the primary carers of children (who today are still primarily women) refuse to do the unpaid labour of childrearing, even for a few hours, others must perform those activities instead and social awareness can profoundly shift. From Iceland, Poland and Spain, to South America, the US and beyond, women and non-binary people have taken strike action in recent years from both paid and unpaid work, and they have done so with powerful demands pertaining to gender-based violence, pay equity, abortion bans, the closing of public services and more again.[50] A coordinated global movement has developed around these mobilisations: the International Women's Strike movement actively supports and facilitates women's strikes across a wide range of countries.[51] As scholars and activists have emphasised, strikes of this kind are strategically important as they demonstrate 'the enormous political potential of women's power: *the power of those whose paid and unpaid work sustains the world*.[52] They also help to build solidarity across oppressed and exploited groups, and highlight the wide range of issues – well beyond those normally considered workplace concerns – which are intimately embroiled in women's working lives: not only wages, hours and on-call allowances, but 'sexual harassment and assault, barriers to reproductive justice, and curbs on the right to strike'.[53] It is notoriously difficult for birth workers to take strike action, and not least in current conditions where back-up – and therefore care for people in labour – is in such short supply. Yet that is precisely why strike action of this kind is so needed. In this respect I am reminded of one of the most powerful slogans I know: 'A Women's Strike is impossible; that is why it is necessary.'[54] Whether impossible or not, I sometimes wonder how many midwives, doulas and birth workers are involved in the Women's Strike social movement, and if so, the kinds of demands, conversations and relationships of solidarity they are making and gestating.

Birth workers have a range of skills and understandings that are profoundly pertinent for the building and nurturing of futures in which the oppressions and exploitations of the present no longer predominate. Much of the work of midwifery, at least when unconstrained by hospital regulations, understaffing and assembly-line labour processes, focuses upon the building of strong and trusting relationships – relations of communality even. Even the words used to signify birth attendants and midwives often gesture towards the kinds of relationality that underpin much of their work and commitments. In Aotearoa New Zealand, Naomi Simmonds explains that the word kaiwhakawhānau (birth attendant) translates from the Māori language into the English language as 'she/he who facilitates the creation of whānau'.[55] In the words of Māori scholar Christine Kenney, the very role of kaiwhakawhānau is to 'facilitate the creation and development of whānau'.[56] When birth care centres the support and development of whānau, profoundly communal relations are being nurtured and supported.[57] The word 'midwife' derives from the old English of pre-capitalist times, in which *mid* broadly meant *with*. The original sense of the word appears to have been 'a woman who is with the mother'.[58] Given such etymology, the work of midwifery is often interpreted as being 'with woman'. That was certainly the case in the north of England amidst the traditions which shaped my own understandings of birth from an early age. Today, I still consider midwifery practices of being *with* women as they bear children to be powerful and important, and I would add to this the practices of midwives being *with* non-binary pregnant people, with childbearing men, with childbearing people's extended kinship/friendship networks, etc. So often when birthing is traumatic, a birth worker has not had the time or inclination to develop connections with the childbearing person and their birth supporter/s (to *be with* them so to speak). 'Being with' does not mean taking away somebody else's pain. 'Being with' involves the development of relations of trust within and through which people can determine the conditions of their own labours. 'Being with' is decidedly *not* 'conveyor-belt' care. It is far more akin to the building of solidarity, than to the dynamics of subsumption.

People draw upon a range of histories and traditions as they reflect on the creation of futures which circumvent the coercions and exploitations of the present. Given my own history, I often take inspiration from the notion of 'being *with*' that I associate with the word midwife. 'Being with' might be considered an approach, a particular modulation or inflection even, of *care*. It might understood as a tonality of care that has always had more than one expression but that is in danger of being lost in birthing places where risk, algorithms and the mechanics of productivity command more space and time than do birthing people and those they love. Simple acts and practices of care – of 'being with', for instance – are frequently neglected amidst the intensities and demands of contemporary capitalism, and that has not been unobserved by many contemporary writers and activists. We need 'promiscuous care', wrote the collective authors of *The Care Manifesto* in 2020.[59] That is to say, 'caring *more* and in ways that remain experimental and extensive by current standards'.[60] Lynne Segal suggests that the caring expected of mothers is increasingly difficult to perform in contemporary conditions, not least because of the exacting demands of paid and precarious employment.[61] She advocates embedding 'mothering at the heart of politics', thereby creating the conditions in which people – be they biological parents or not – can care for whomever needs that support.[62] Reflecting the vast numbers of people and carers across the world, and the diversity of their histories, there will be many more approaches to the creation of social formations which take care seriously. Intonations of 'being with' are just one suggestion.

As I reflect on the possibilities of worlds in which relations of oppression and exploitation have been interrupted, and perhaps even replaced by relations of care and support, I find myself contemplating how childbirth might be approached in such contexts. My ruminations around this are not overly expansive, particularly because the birthing landscapes that are most needed must respond to the specific needs of birthing people and their communities as *they* define them. Local and historical conditions shape what is necessary, what is needed, what is possible and what is not. Given that caveat, I long for the so-called 'time-consuming' aspects of birth work – of supporting, caring and just 'being there' – to be valued and nurtured. Perhaps birth workers will be accountable to their people via collectively (and locally) determined arrangements which do not engender debilitating fear. I unreservedly hope that the care needs of people with birth injuries will be met without legal battles to prove clinical negligence. Babies will not be born in prisons, and adults will not be held there either. Racism, colonialism, sexism, homophobia, transphobia and ableism are incompatible with the futures I long for. I hope that technologies will be created and used for human and planetary benefit rather than profit, and I anticipate that science will assume a range of exciting expressions – it already does. I long for the building of health and well-being to displace the frenzied identification and impossible closure of risk. Some of the developments for which I most hope are already happening – at least in places and at least in part. Many people are already working hard to create, and therefore recreate, ways of caring that are culturally safe for all. Futures are not delivered by the stork. They grow from the determinations, imaginations and possibilities of the present …

At times, the birthing of futures less marked than today by exploitation and oppression, appear closer than at others. Some years after the 2008 financial crisis, various political developments suggested that tides might be turning, that contractions (emergent contradictions even) might be gathering pace. There were uprisings across Arab nations, and the development of political movements in Greece, Spain and even in England that appeared firmly committed to tackling poverty and challenging inequality. The Black Lives Matter movement gathered global momentum. In so far as birth is concerned, I sensed growing hope for change when midwives and nurses in a range of countries 'downed tools' and demonstrated in the streets, demanding their work and therefore public safety be taken seriously. Various developments including, but not limited to, the long duration of a pandemic, have substantially altered local and global dynamics. While I am emboldened by the possibility that the groundswell of support for the Palestinian people might be growing, the far right is gaining ground, and rapidly so in some parts of the world. Weather- and climate-related disasters are on the rise.[63] Today, I sometimes struggle to feel optimistic about the short-term prospects for substantial social change oriented towards equity and social justice. But progress – if we can use that word at all in relation to either childbirth or society – is far from linear. In seeking to navigate the contemporary political-economic milieu, I am reminded of the retroactive ways in which people make sense of their own experiences of giving birth. Some people revisit specific moments of parturition over and again in their minds, until those make sense in ways that they did not before. It was well after I had given birth for the last time, that I began to understand the hardest pain and transitory panic that I experienced during that labour, as marking the moment of transition. In birthing spaces, the word 'transition' tends to denote a time shortly before someone begins to push the baby that they hold so intimately within their bodies, into the 'outside' world. Involved is a shift in physiological processes that can be profoundly disorientating and intensely painful. It was only in retrospect, months after the event, that I could script for myself that moment of transition in my own labour. It was followed shortly after by the indescribable experience of holding and cradling a very new person in my arms. I sometimes wonder if we will ever be able to look back and identify, to return to Marx's words, the 'prolonged birth pangs' which preceded the emergence of a post-capitalist society.[64] To deny the possibility of transitioning to non-capitalist modes of production, profoundly naturalises a political-economic system that has predominated for little more than two, perhaps three, hundred years. Regardless of what the future holds, attempts to challenge the relations of exploitation and violence which currently predominate, can hardly be wasted. Such ventures, such collective pushes, might even enable the growth and flourishing of more solidarity and shared political understanding – more 'being with', more energies directed towards justice and equity – in the present, while also preparing the way for futures that may yet emerge.

Glossary

Definitions for some of the terms used in this book vary. This glossary is intended only as an introductory guide.

Active management of labour A set of procedures and protocols developed by obstetrician Dr. Kieran O'Driscoll to manage the labour of childbirth. See Chapter 3 for more details.

Antenatal During pregnancy (before birth).

Epidural analgesia (often called an epidural) A form of analgesia used during labour that affects sensation in the lower part of the body (primarily between the belly button and upper legs). The doctor who puts an epidural in place is called an anaesthetist (anesthesiologist in the US). A small catheter (tube) is inserted into the epidural space (which is close to the childbearing person's spinal cord) and pain-relieving drugs are passed through the catheter.

Episiotomy A surgical cut to a birthing person's perineum to widen the opening of the vagina and expedite the birth of the baby. In the past, episiotomies have been performed relatively routinely in many maternity hospitals. It is now considered best practice that episiotomies are only carried out in very specific clinical circumstances.

Forceps Curved surgical instruments that are sometimes used to facilitate the birth of a baby. The forceps are placed around the baby's head, and when the birthing person has a contraction, the obstetrician pulls with sufficient traction to encourage the birth of the baby.

Induction of labour Deliberate procedures and practices aimed at encouraging the labour (of childbirth) to begin. In this book, the term is used in reference to pharmacological and/or surgical methods aimed at stimulating labour to start, and the use of mechanical methods such as insertion of a balloon catheter (an inflatable catheter) into the pregnant person's cervix (the opening of their uterus).

Instrumental birth A birth in which ventouse suction (sometimes called vacuum extraction) or forceps are used.

Maternal death In broad terms, the death of a person while they are pregnant, in labour, or during the period that follows. Definitions of, and methods for measuring, maternal mortality have varied historically and geographically. The World Health Organization currently defines maternal deaths as 'female deaths from any cause related to or aggravated by pregnancy or its management (excluding accidental or incidental causes) during pregnancy and childbirth or within 42 days of termination of pregnancy, irrespective of the duration and site of the pregnancy'.[1]

Neonatal Pertaining to the first month of a baby's life. According to the World Health Organization, 'The neonatal period begins with birth and ends 28 complete days after birth.'[2]

Neonatal death Defined by the World Health Organization as '[d]eath after birth and within the first 28 days of life'.[3]

Perinatal In broad terms, the period around birth. Precise definitions vary.

Perinatal mortality Deaths of newborn babies and of foetuses beyond a specific gestational age. Precise definitions vary. The World Health Organization currently defines perinatal mortality as 'the number of fetal deaths of at least 28 weeks of gestation and/or 1000 g in weight *and* newborn deaths (up to and including the first seven days after birth)'.[4]

Ventouse A cup-shaped suction device that, in specific circumstances during labour, is attached to the baby's head by an obstetrician (or a specifically trained midwife) and used to assist the birth of the baby.

Notes

CHAPTER 1 CONCEIVING CHILDBIRTH

1. Denis Campbell, 'Midwives to Strike after Jeremy Hunt Scraps 1% Pay Rise', *Guardian*, 29 September 2014, www.theguardian.com/society/2014/sep/29/midwives-strike-over-1-percent-pay-rise-first-in-history (last accessed April 2024).
2. See, for instance, Kate Gregan and Sam Olley, '"We're All Burning out": Auckland, Northland Midwives Start Rolling Strikes', *Radio New Zealand*, 9 August 2021, www.rnz.co.nz/news/national/448830/we-re-all-burning-out-auckland-northland-midwives-start-rolling-strikes (last accessed April 2024); Don Rowe, 'March of the Midwives', *The Spinoff*, 3 May 2018, https://thespinoff.co.nz/parenting/03-05-2018/march-of-the-midwives/ (last accessed April 2024); 'Nurses Gather Nationwide to Protest Over Staff Shortages, Pay and Conditions', *Radio New Zealand*, 15 April 2023, www.rnz.co.nz/news/national/488003/nurses-gather-nationwide-to-protest-over-staff-shortages-pay-and-conditions (last accessed April 2024).
3. Penny Curtis, Linda Ball and Mavis Kirkham, 'Why Do Midwives Leave? (Not) Being the Kind of Midwife You Want to Be', *British Journal of Midwifery* 14, no. 1 (2006): 27–31; Royal College of Midwives, *Why Midwives Leave – Revisited* (UK: Royal College of Midwives, October 2016). https://cdn.ps.emap.com/wp-content/uploads/sites/3/2016/10/Why-Midwives-Leave.pdf (last accessed April 2024).
4. See, for example, Alison Young, 'Deadly Deliveries: A USA TODAY Investigation', *USA Today*, 22 March 2021, www.usatoday.com/story/news/investigations/2021/03/22/deadly-deliveries-usa-today-investigation/4802861001 (last accessed April 2024); Alissa Erogbogbo, 'The US is the Second-most Expensive Country to Give Birth In — Here's What You'll Pay and Tips to Save', *Business Insider*, 1 December 2022, https://tinyurl.com/mrx832fu (last accessed April 2024).
5. Emily Harris, 'US Maternal Mortality Continues to Worsen', *JAMA* 329, no. 15 (March 2023): 1248; Roosa Tikkanen, Munira Z. Gunja, Molly FitzGerald and Laurie C. Zephyrin, 'Maternal Mortality and Maternity Care in the United States Compared to 10 Other Developed Countries', *The Commonwealth Fund*, 18 November 2020, www.commonwealthfund.org/publications/issue-briefs/2020/nov/maternal-mortality-maternity-care-us-compared-10-countries (last accessed January 2024).
6. Donna L. Hoyert, 'Maternal Mortality Rates in the United States, 2021', NCHS Health E-Stats (2023). https://dx.doi.org/10.15620/cdc:124678; For discussion of debates around the accuracy of the US maternal mortality data, see Robin Fields, 'What to Know about the Roiling Debate over U.S. Maternal Mortality

Rates', *ProPublica*, 5 April 2024. www.propublica.org/article/what-to-know-maternal-mortality-rates-debate (last accessed April 2024).

7. S. Leitao, E. Manning, R.A. Greene and P. Corcoran, 'On Behalf of the Maternal Morbidity Advisory Group. Maternal Morbidity and Mortality: An Iceberg Phenomenon', *BJOG* 129 (2022): 402–411.
8. World Health Organization, *Born Too Soon: Decade of Action on Preterm Birth* (Geneva: World Health Organization, 2023).
9. Mary J. Renfrew, Elena Ateva, Jemima Araba Dennis-Antwi, Deborah Davis, Lesley Dixon, Peter Johnson, Holly Powell Kennedy, Anneka Knutsson, Ornella Lincetto, Fran McConville, Alison McFadden, Hatsumi Taniguchi, Petra Ten Hoope Bender and Willibald Zeck, 'Midwifery is a Vital Solution—What is Holding Back Global Progress?', *Birth* 46, no. 3 (2019): 396–399
10. Examples include, but are far from limited to, Barbara Katz Rothman, *Recreating Motherhood: Ideology and Technology in a Patriarchal Society*, (New York & London: W. W. Norton & Company, 1989), 65–81; Elizabeth Newnham, Lois McKellar and Jan Pincombe, *Towards the Humanisation of Birth: A Study of Epidural Analgesia and Hospital Birth Culture* (Palgrave Macmillan, 2018); Diana Russell, 'Control of Childbirth: A Socialist Feminist Perspective', *Nursing Praxis in New Zealand*, 5, no. 3 (July 1990): 12–17.
11. Mavis Kirkham, 'Midwives Should – Change It' *Midwifery Matters* 180 (2024): 28–29.
12. Raymond Williams, *Politics and Letters: Interviews with New Left Review*, (London: New Left Books, 1979), 146–147.
13. 'A Neglected Global Crisis for Women: Nearly 300,000 Mothers Died in 2020 from Preventable Causes', *UNFPA*, 24 February 2023. https://tinyurl.com/4e7yvcnx (last accessed April 2024).
14. 'Caesarean Section Rates Continue to Rise, amid Growing Inequalities in Access', *World Health Organization*, 16 June 2021, https://tinyurl.com/eus8krek (last accessed April 2024).
15. Jane Sandall, Rachel M. Tribe, Lisa Avery, Glen Mola, Gerard Ha Visser, Caroline Se Homer, Deena Gibbons, Niamh M Kelly, Holly Powell Kennedy, Hussein Kidanto, Paul Taylor and Marleen Temmerman, 'Short-Term and Long-Term Effects of Caesarean Section on the Health of Women and Children', *The Lancet* 392, no. 10155 (October 2018): 1349–1357.
16. Olufemi T. Oladapo, Mustafa A. Lamina and Adewale O Sule-Odu, 'Maternal Morbidity and Mortality Associated with Elective Caesarean Delivery at a University Hospital in Nigeria', *Australian and New Zealand Journal of Obstetrics and Gynaecology*, 47 (2007): 110–114; Maleda Tefera, Nega Assefa, Bezatu Mengistie, Aklilu Abrham, Kedir Teji and Teshager Worku, 'Elective Cesarean Section on Term Pregnancies Has a High Risk for Neonatal Respiratory Morbidity in Developed Countries: A Systematic Review and Meta-Analysis', *Frontiers in Pediatrics* 8, no. 286 (25 June 2020), doi:10.3389/fped.2020.00286; Newton Opiyo, Saverio Bellizzi, Maria Regina Torloni, Joao Paulo Souza and Ana Pilar Betran, 'Association Between Prelabour Caesarean Section and Perinatal Outcomes: Analysis of Demographic and Health Surveys from 26 Low-Income and Middle-Income Countries', *BMJ Open* 12, no. 1 (1 January 2022), doi:10.1136/bmjopen-2021-053049

17. Suellen Miller, Edgardo Abalos, Monica Chamillard, Agustin Ciapponi, Daniela Colaci, Daniel Comandé, Virginia Diaz, Stacie Geller, Claudia Hanson, Ana Langer, Victoria Manuelli, Kathryn Millar, Imran Morhason-Bello, Cynthia Pileggi Castro, Vicky Nogueira Pileggi, Nuriya Robinson, Michelle Skaer, João Paulo Souza, Joshua P. Vogel and Fernando Althabe, 'Beyond Too Little, Too Late and Too Much, Too Soon: A Pathway towards Evidence-Based, Respectful Maternity Care Worldwide.' *The Lancet* 388, no. 10056 (29 October 2016): 2176–2192.
18. Marjorie Tew, *Safer Childbirth? A Critical History of Maternity Care*. (England: Chapman and Hall [E-book], 1990), 32.
19. Irvine Loudon, 'Deaths in Childbed from the Eighteenth Century to 1935,' *Medical History* 30, no. 1 (1986): 3–6.
20. Data from 'Reports of the Registrar General' and 'On the state of the Public Health', cited in Loudon, 'Deaths in Childbed from the Eighteenth Century to 1935', 3.
21. Loudon, 'Deaths in Childbed from the Eighteenth Century to 1935', 6.
22. Irvine Loudon, 'Maternal Mortality in the Past and Its Relevance to Developing Countries Today', *American Journal of Clinical Nutrition* 72, no. 1 (1 July 2000): 243S & 246S.
23. Loudon, 'Maternal Mortality in the Past, 242S–243S.
24. Loudon, 'Deaths in Childbed from the Eighteenth Century to 1935', 3.
25. Tew, *Safer Childbirth? A Critical History of Maternity Care*, 216.
26. Lauren A. Plante, 'Mommy, What Did You Do in the Industrial Revolution? Meditations on the Rising Cesarean Rate', *International Journal of Feminist Approaches to Bioethics* 2, no. 1 (2009): 140–147; Michel Odent, *Childbirth in the Age of Plastics* (London: Pinter & Martin Ltd., 2011), 87–93.
27. Heather A. Cahill, 'Male Appropriation and Medicalization of Childbirth: An Historical Analysis', *Journal of Advanced Nursing* 33, no. 3 (2001): 334–342.
28. Jean Donnison, *Midwives and Medical Men: A History of the Struggle for the Control of Childbirth*, 2nd ed. (Herts & London: Historical Publications, 1988): 67, 176 & 34.
29. Te Ahukaramū Charles Royal, 'Papatūānuku – the land', *Te Ara – the Encyclopedia of New Zealand*, www.teara.govt.nz/en/papatuanuku-the-land/page-1 (last accessed May 2024).
30. Te Ahukaramū Charles Royal, 'Papatūānuku – the Land – Whenua – the Placenta', *Te Ara – the Encyclopedia of New Zealand*, https://teara.govt.nz/en/papatuanuku-the-land/page-4 (last accessed May 2024); Dianne Wepa and Jean Te Huia observe that there are variations in how whenua ki te whenua is practiced: Wepa and Te Huia, 'Cultural Safety and the Birth Culture of Maori', *Social Work Review* 18, no. 2 (2006): 26–31, 26.
31. In the words of Suzanne Miller and Teresa Krishnan, 'The whenua is returned to Papatūānuku to nurture her as she has nurtured both the wahine [woman] and pēpi thoughout the hapūtanga [pregnancy] journey': Miller and Krishnan, 'Whakawhanaungatanga – Making Families; The Sociocultural Politics of Birthspace Design', in *The Politics of Design: Privilege and Prejudice in Aotearoa New Zealand, Australia and South Africa*, eds Federico Freschi, Jane Venis and Farieda Nazier (Dunedin, New Zealand: Otago Polytechnic Press, 2021): 211–228, 220.

32. Annie Mikaere, 'Māori Women: Caught in the Contradictions of a Colonised Reality', *Waikato Law Review* 2 (1994): 125-149, especially 133–142.
33. See, for example, Wepa and Te Huia, 'Cultural Safety and the Birth Culture of Maori', 28–29.
34. Miller and Krishnan, 'Whakawhanaungatanga – Making Families', 221–222; Naomi Simmonds, 'Honouring Our Ancestors: Reclaiming the Power of Māori Maternities', in *Indigenous Experiences of Pregnancy and Birth*, eds Hannah Tait Neufeld and Jaime Cidro (Ontario, Canada: Demeter Press, 2017) 111–28, 119.
35. Marian Knight, Kathryn Bunch, Allison Felker, Roshni Patel, Rohit Kotnis, Sara Kenyon and Jennifer J. Kurinczuk, eds on behalf of MBRRACE-UK, *Saving Lives, Improving Mothers' Care Core Report – Lessons learned to inform maternity care from the UK and Ireland Confidential Enquiries into Maternal Deaths and Morbidity 2019–21* (Oxford: National Perinatal Epidemiology Unit, University of Oxford 2023).
36. Emily E. Petersen, Nicole L. Davis, David Goodman, Shanna Cox, Carla Syverson, Kristi Seed, Carrie Shapiro-Mendoza, William M. Callaghan and Wanda Barfield. 'Racial/Ethnic Disparities in Pregnancy-Related Deaths — United States, 2007–2016', *Morbidity and Mortality Weekly Report* 68, no. 35 (2019): 762–765.
37. 'Maternal Mortality and Severe Maternal Morbidity Surveillance', *City of New York, NYC Health*, www.nyc.gov/site/doh/data/data-sets/maternal-morbidity-mortality-surveillance.page (last accessed April 2024).
38. Sezin Topçu and Patrick Brown, 'Editorial: The Impact of Technology on Pregnancy and Childbirth: Creating and Managing Obstetrical Risk in Different Cultural and Socio-Economic Contexts', *Health, Risk & Society* 21, no. 3–4 (19 May 2019): 89–99, 97.
39. Cecilia Benoit, Maria Zadoroznyj, Helga Hallgrimsdottir, Adrienne Treloar and Kara Taylor, 'Medical Dominance and Neoliberalisation in Maternal Care Provision: The Evidence from Canada and Australia', *Social Science & Medicine* 71, no. 3 (2010): 475–481 , 477–478.
40. Barbara Bridgman Perkins, *The Medical Delivery Business: Health Reform, Childbirth, and the Economic Order* (New Brunswick, NJ: Rutgers University Press, 2003), 7.
41. Jennie Joseph, 'Midwife Jennie Joseph: Saving Ourselves from a Capitalist Medical System (an edited transcript)', *Kindred Media*, 7 April 2018. www.kindredmedia.org/2018/04/midwife-jennie-joseph/
42. Ibid.
43. See, for example, Christine McCourt and Fiona Dykes, 'From Tradition to Modernity: Time and Childbirth in Historical Perspective', in *Childbirth, Midwifery and Concepts of Time*, ed. Christine McCourt (Berghahn Books, ebook edition, 2013).
44. Sally K. Tracy, 'Costing Birth as Commodity or Sustainable Public Good'. In: *Sustainability, Midwifery and Birth*, eds Lorna Davies, Rea Daellenbach and Mary Kensington (London and New York: Routledge, 2nd ed., 2021), 31–64, 34.
45. Ibid., 34.
46. For one aspect of such a conversation, see Rebecca Ashley, 'Contraction II: Crisis with Rebecca Ashley', *Contractions: The Politics of Midwifery* (produced by Rodante van der Waal and Vinny Taylor), 15 December 2020, https://

contractions.buzzsprout.com/677121/6855679-contraction-ii-crisis-with-rebecca-ashley (last accessed May 2024).

47. Ellen Meiksins Wood, *The Origin of Capitalism: A Longer View* (Verso, Kindle Edition), 20.
48. Ibid., 9.
49. Karl Marx, *Capital, Vol. 1*, trans. Ben Fowkes (Penguin Books, 1976); Karl Marx, *Capital, Vol. 2*, trans. David Fernbach (Penguin Books, 1976).
50. Karl Marx and Friedrich Engels, *The Communist Manifesto* (Penguin Books, 2002), 225.
51. Ernest Mandel, *Power and Money* (London and New York: Verso, 1992), 159.
52. For a closely related discussion regarding the return to a focus upon capitalism within theory and activism, see Nancy Fraser, 'Behind Marx's Hidden Abode: For an Expanded Conception of Capitalism', *New Left Review* 86 (March–April 2014): 55–72.
53. Fredric Jameson, 'Postmodernism, or The Cultural Logic of Late Capitalism', *New Left Review*, 146 (1984): 53–92, 77.
54. Barbara Katz Rothman, 'Laboring Then: The Political History of Maternity Care in the United States', in *Laboring On: Birth in Transition in the United States*, eds Wendy Simonds, Barbara Katz Rothman and Bari Meltzer Norman (Routledge, 2007), 3–28, 19.
55. Katz Rothman, 'Laboring Then', 19.
56. Grantly Dick-Reed, *Childbirth Without Fear* (London: William Heinemann Medical Books Ltd., 1958 [3rd edition]), 230.
57. Barbara Katz Rothman wrote of finding the term 'prepared childbirth' more useful in the context of US hospitals. 'Laboring Then', 19.
58. Ann Oakley, 'Social Consequences of Obstetric Technology: The Importance of Measuring "Soft" Outcomes', *Birth* 10, no. 2 (Summer 1983): 99–108, 107.
59. See, for instance, Jessica Grose, 'Welcome to NYT Parenting: Here's Why We Won't Say "Natural Birth"', *New York Times*, 7 May 2019, https://tinyurl.com/bddtspp6 (last accessed June 2024).
60. Markella Rutherford and Selina Gallo-Cruz, 'Selling the Ideal Birth: Rationalisation and Re-Enchantment in the Marketing of Maternity Care' in *Patients, Consumers and Civil Society*, eds Susan M. Chambré and Melinda Goldner (Bingley, UK: Emerald, JAI, 2008), 75–98, 92–93.
61. Rutherford and Gallo-Cruz, 'Selling the Ideal Birth', 93.
62. Marcy Darnovsky, 'Be Wary of the Techno-Fix', in *Once and Future Feminist*, ed. Merve Emre (Cambridge, MA: Boston Review/Boston Critic Inc., 2018), 48–52, 49.
63. Karl Marx, *Grundrisse*, trans. Martin Nicolaus (Penguin Books, 1973), 100.
64. Ibid.
65. Ibid.
66. Karl Marx, *A Contribution to The Critique Of The Political Economy*, trans. N.I. Stone (e-artnow, 2019): 146.
67. David Harvey, 'History versus Theory: A Commentary on Marx's Method in Capital', *Historical Materialism* 20, no. 2 (2012): 3–38, 10.
68. Alberto Toscano, 'The Culture of Abstraction', *Theory, Culture & Society* 25, no. 4 (2008): 57–75.
69. Darnovsky, 'Be Wary of the Techno-Fix', 49.

70. 'The machine that goes PING!', 'The Miracle of Birth' scene from *Monty Python's Meaning of Life* (1983), available at www.youtube.com/watch?v=_YruT2ROEUc
71. Barbara Katz Rothman, 'Editorial: Pregnancy, Birth and Risk – an Introduction', *Health, Risk & Society* 16, no. 1 (2 January 2014): 1–6, 1.
72. Sophie Lewis, *Full Surrogacy Now: Feminism against Family* (Verso, 2019), 5.
73. Eugene R. Declercq, Carol Sakala, Maureen P. Corry, Sandra Applebaum and Ariel Herrlich, *Listening to Mothers SM III: Pregnancy and Birth* (New York: Childbirth Connection, May 2013), 24–25.
74. Ann Oakley, 'The Sociology of Childbirth: An Autobiographical Journey through Four Decades of Research', *Sociology of Health & Illness* 38, no. 5 (1 June 2016): 689–705, 695–696.
75. Carol Sakala, Eugene R. Declercq, Jessica M. Turon and Maureen P. Corry, *Listening to Mothers in California: A Population-Based Survey of Women's Childbearing Experiences, Full Survey Report* (Washington, DC: National Partnership for Women and Families, 2018), 32.
76. Sakala et al., *Listening to Mothers in California*, 52.
77. Archie Cochrane, *Effectiveness and Efficiency: Random Reflections on Health Services* (England: The Nuffield Provincial Hospitals Trust, 1972), 5–6.
78. A.L. Cochrane, '1931–1971: A Critical Review with Particular Reference to the Medical Profession', in *Medicines for the Year 2000: A Symposium Held at the Royal College of Physicians, London in September 1978 by the Office of Health Economics*, eds George Teeling-Smith and Nicola Wells (London: Office of Health Economics, 1979), 2–12, 11.
79. Ibid.
80. Ibid.
81. Sarah Donovan, 'Inescapable Burden of Choice? The Impact of a Culture of Prenatal Screening on Women's Experiences of Pregnancy', *Health Sociology Review* 15, no. 4 (2006): 397–405.
82. Blake Gutt, 'Medieval Trans Lives in Anamorphosis: Looking Back and Seeing Differently (Pregnant Men and Backward Birth)', *Medieval Feminist Forum* 55, no. 1 (2019): 174–206; Kassie Hartendorp, 'What Do We Really Know about Gender Diversity in Te Ao Māori?', *The Spinoff*, 23 October 2019, https://thespinoff.co.nz/atea/23-10-2019/what-do-we-really-know-about-gender-diversity-in-te-ao-maori/. (last accessed April 2024).
83. This particular section of *The Midwives Act* continued: 'any woman so acting without being certified under this Act shall be liable on summary conviction to a fine not exceeding ten pounds, provided this section shall not apply to legally qualified medical practitioners, or to any one rendering assistance in a case of emergency': 'The Midwives Act', 1. (2), *British Medical Journal* 2, no. 2172 (1902): 481–483, 481.
84. Holly Lewis, *The Politics of Everybody: Feminism, Queer Theory and Marxism at the Intersection* (London: Zed Books, 2016), 126.
85. See, for example, Rachel Holmes, *The Secret Life of Dr James Barry: Victorian England's Most Eminent Surgeon* (Bloomsbury Publishing, 2020).
86. Lewis, *The Politics of Everybody*, 104.
87. See, for example, Rachel Aldred, 'In Perspective – Judith Butler', *International Socialism* 103 (2004), http://isj.org.uk/in-perspective-judith-butler/ (last accessed April 2024); Endnotes, 'The Logic of Gender', *Endnotes* 3, September

2013, https://endnotes.org.uk/translations/endnotes-the-logic-of-gender (last accessed April 2024).
88. Aldred, 'In Perspective – Judith Butler'.
89. Judith Butler, 'Contingent Foundations: Feminism and the Question of 'Postmodernism'', in *Feminists Theorize the Political*, eds Judith Butler and Joan W. Scott (Routledge, 1992), 3–21, 17.
90. Judith Butler, *Gender Trouble: Feminism and the Subversion of Identity* (Routledge, 1990), 6.
91. Ibid.
92. See Endnotes, 'The Logic of Gender'.
93. See, for example, Loretta Ross and Rickie Solinger, *Reproductive Justice: An Introduction* (Oakland: University of California Press, 2017, Kindle Edition), 8.
94. George Christy Parker, 'Mothers at Large: Governing Fat Pregnant Embodiment' (Doctor of Philosophy in Sociology Thesis, University of Auckland, 2019), 19.
95. 'whānau' in *Te Aka Māori-English, English-Māori Dictionary*, (Auckland: Pearson, 2011), 257.
96. In the words of George Parker, Elizabeth Kerekere, Fleur Kelsey and Suzanne Miller, 'A whānau-centred approach to midwifery care asks midwives to invite the pregnant person to share who and what is significant to them and to provide care that is responsive to the self-determined needs and aspirations of each whānau.' 'Cutting Through the Noise: Why Whānau-Centred Midwifery is Not Erasing Women', *The Spinoff*, 1 March 2024, https://thespinoff.co.nz/society/01-03-2024/cutting-through-the-noise-why-whanau-centred-midwifery-is-not-erasing-women (last accessed May 2024).

CHAPTER 2 STRETCH MARX

1. Karl Marx and Frederick Engels, *The German Ideology* (London: Lawrence & Wishart, 1965), 39, 41.
2. Ibid., 41.
3. Ibid.
4. Frederick Engels, 'Preface to the First Edition' of *The Origin of the Family, Private Property and the State* (London: Lawrence & Wishart, 1972), 71.
5. Marx & Engels, *The German Ideology*, 41.
6. See, for example, Maria Mies, *Patriarchy and Accumulation on a World Scale: Women in the International Division of Labour* (London: Zed Books, 2014).
7. Karl Marx, 'Author's Preface' to *A Contribution to The Critique Of The Political Economy*, trans. N.I. Stone (e-artnow, 2019), paragraph 4.
8. Karl Marx, *Capital, Volume 1*, trans. Ben Fowkes (Penguin Books, 1976), 916.
9. Sheila Rowbotham, *Women, Resistance and Revolution: A History of Women and Revolution in the Modern World* (Verso, Ebook edition, 2014), 58.
10. Frantz Fanon, *The Wretched of the Earth*, trans. Constance Farrington (New York: Grove Press, 1963), 40.
11. Ibid., 40.
12. Ibid., 40.
13. See discussion of some of these movements, which include strands of feminism and of anti-colonial struggle, in Silvia Federici, *Re-Enchanting the World: Feminism and the Politics of the Commons* (Oakland, CA: PM Press, 2019). In

the same text, Federici also cites, in a footnote, the aforementioned words by Fanon (169, footnote 8).

14. Fanon, *The Wretched of the Earth*, 278.
15. Marx, *Capital, Vol. 1*, 718.
16. Susan Ferguson and David McNally, 'Capital, Labour-Power, and Gender-Relations: Introduction to the Historical Materialism Edition of Marxism and the Oppression of Women', in Lise Vogel, *Marxism and the Oppression of Women*, (Leiden & Boston, MA: Brill, 2013), xvii–xl, xxvii.
17. Ferguson and McNally, 'Capital, Labour-Power, and Gender-Relations', xxvii.
18. In the words of Martha Gimenez, 'to me, this claim meant that capitalists are indifferent to the workers' fate *except when it may impinge on their own safety and ability to accumulate*.' *Marx, Women, and Capitalist Social Reproduction* (Leiden & Boston: Brill, 2019), 294; original emphasis.
19. Marx, *Capital, Vol. 1*, 718.
20. See Georgina Murray, 'Australia's Ruling Class: A Local Elite, a Transnational Capitalist Class or Bits of Both?', in *Financial Elites and Transnational Business: Who Rules the World?* eds Georgina Murray and John Scott (Cheltenham, UK: Edward Elgar, 2012), 193–219, 198–199.
21. Karl Marx, *Capital, Vol. 2*, trans. David Fernbach (Penguin Books, 1976), 109.
22. Ibid., 109.
23. Ibid., 110.
24. Tithi Bhattacharya, 'How Not to Skip Class: Social Reproduction of Labour and the Global Working Class', in *Social Reproduction Theory: Remapping Class, Recentering Oppression*, ed. Tithi Bhattacharya (London: Pluto Press, 2017), 68–93, 81.
25. Marx, *Capital, Vol. 1*, 717.
26. Ibid., 718.
27. Ibid., 795.
28. Ibid., 844.
29. These words are from an 1864 Public Health Report quoted by Marx in the footnotes of *Capital, Vol. 1*, 837 (n97).
30. Ibid..
31. Frederick Engels, *The Condition of the Working Class in England* (Moscow & London: Progress Publishers; Lawrence & Wishart, 1973), 175.
32. Ibid.
33. Lisa Forman Cody, 'Living and Dying in Georgian London's Lying-In Hospitals', *Bulletin of the History of Medicine* 78, no. 2 (15 June 2004): 309–48, 313.
34. Alexandra Kollontai, 'Working Woman and Mother', in *Selected Writings of Alexandra Kollontai*, ed. & trans. Alix Holt (Westport, CT: Lawrence Hill & Company, 1978), 127–39, 127.
35. Ibid., 130.
36. Ibid.
37. Ibid.
38. Ibid.
39. Ibid.
40. Ibid., 131.
41. Ibid., 133.
42. Engels, *The Condition of the Working Class in England*, 175.

43. Ibid.
44. Ibid., 176.
45. Susan Ferguson, *Women and Work: Feminism, Labour and Social Reproduction* (London: Pluto Press, 2020), 12.
46. Ferguson, *Women and Work*, 13.
47. Kollontai, 'Working Woman and Mother', 133.
48. Engels, *The Condition of the Working Class in England*, 161.
49. Engels describes these words as testimonies from working women that were presented by Lord Ashley to the House of Commons in 1844. Cited in Engels, *The Condition of the Working Class in England*, 161.
50. Marx, *Capital, Vol. 1*, 521.
51. Ibid., 521. See also 517–518 (fn 38).
52. Ibid., 518 (fn 39).
53. For a non-Marxist history of this, see Rima D. Apple, '"Advertised by Our Loving Friends": The Infant Formula Industry and the Creation of New Pharmaceutical Markets, 1870–1910', *Journal of the History of Medicine and Allied Sciences* 41, no. 1 (1986): 3–23.
54. Marx, *Capital, Vol. 1*, 875.
55. Ibid., 876.
56. 'So-called primitive accumulation, therefore, is nothing else than the historical process of divorcing the producer from the means of production. It appears as "primitive" because it forms the pre-history of capital, and of the mode of production corresponding to capital': Ibid., 874–875.
57. Terry Eagleton, *Why Marx Was Right* (New Haven, CT and London: Yale University Press, 2018), 181–182.
58. Marx, *Capital, Vol. 1*, 915, 931–41.
59. Karl Marx, *The Poverty of Philosophy* (London: Lawrence & Wishart, Martin Lawrence Limited), 94–95.
60. Silvia Federici, *Caliban and the Witch* (Brooklyn, NY: Autonomedia, 2004), 12.
61. Ibid.
62. For such a reading that does not draw on the term 'primitive accumulation', see Barbara Ehrenreich and Deirdre English, *Witches, Midwives, and Nurses: A History of Women Healers* (New York: The Feminist Press, CUNY, 1973).
63. Federici, *Caliban and the Witch*, 88–89.
64. Ibid., 89.
65. Ibid.
66. Ibid.
67. Ibid., 12.
68. Ibid., 220.
69. See, for instance, David McNally, *Monsters of the Market: Zombies, Vampires and Global Capitalism* (Leiden and Boston, MA: Brill, 2011), 45 (fn 74); Joseph Kay, 'Witch-hunts and the Transition to Capitalism?', *libcom.org*, 20 December 2011, https://libcom.org/article/witch-hunts-and-transition-capitalism (last accessed May 2024); From a feminist perspective, see Ann Ferguson, 'Review of Silvia Federici Caliban and the Witch: Women, the Body and Primitive Accumulation (2005, Autonomedia, NYC)', *Wagadu* 3 (Spring 2006): 114–123.
70. See, for instance, Simon Barber, 'Geometries of Life' (PhD dissertation, Goldsmiths, University of London, 2017), including 79–80 and 241–245.

71. Matthew Wynyard, 'Dairying, Dispossession, Devastation: Primitive Accumulation and the New Zealand Dairy Industry, 1814–2018', *Counterfutures* 8 (2019): 10–41, especially 15–16.
72. Ibid., 37–38.
73. Barber, 'Geometries of Life', 271.
74. Cedric J. Robinson, *Black Marxism: The Making of the Black Radical Tradition* (Chapel Hill and London: University of North Carolina Press, 1983), 4.
75. Jennifer L. Morgan and Alys Eve Weinbaum, 'Introduction: Reproductive Racial Capitalism', *History of the Present* 14, no. 1 (April 2024): 1–19, 7.
76. In relation to this, Robinson cites the work and words of Lesley Bethel who notes that in Brazil, in addition to high rates of mortality amongst enslaved people, 'the rate of natural reproduction amongst slaves was extremely low.' Bethel, 'The Independence of Brazil and the Abolition of the Brazilian Slave Trade: Anglo Brazilian Relations, 1822–1826', *Latin American Studies* 1, no. 2 (1969), 118, cited in Robinson, *Black Marxism*, 151.
77. Angela Y. Davis, 'Outcast Mothers and Surrogates: Racism and Reproductive Politics', in *American Feminist Thought at Century's End: A Reader*, ed. Linda Kauffman (Cambridge, MA: Wiley-Blackwell, 1993), 355–366, 356–357.
78. Ibid., 356.
79. Robinson, *Black Marxism*, 2.
80. Claudia Jones, 'An End to the Neglect of the Problems of the Negro Woman!' (Reprinted from 'Political Affairs', by National Women's Commission, C.P.U.S.A., June 1949), 3–19, 5. For a recent discussion of maternal deaths, racism and capitalism in the US, see Deja Gaston, 'US Pregnancy Related Deaths Skyrocket, Capitalism is to Blame', *Liberation*, 13 April 2023 [Initially posted by *Breaking the Chains* Magazine]. www.liberationnews.org/u-s-pregnancy-related-deaths-kkyrocket-capitalism-is-to-blame/ (last accessed April 2024).
81. Jennifer L. Morgan and Alys Eve Weinbaum, 'Introduction: Reproductive Racial Capitalism', *History of the Present* 14 no. 1 (April 2024): 1–19, 2.
82. Marx, *Capital, Volume 1*, 784–794.
83. Ibid., 787. For Engels on Malthus, see *The Condition of the Working Class in England*, 282–284.
84. Angela Y. Davis, *Women, Race and Class* (Penguin, 1981, Kindle Edition).
85. Ibid., 194; original emphasis.
86. Ibid.
87. National Women's Law Center, with help from the Austistic Women and Nonbinary Network, *Forced Sterilization of Disabled People in the USA* (Washington, DC: National Women's Law Centre, 2022), https://nwlc.org/resource/forced-sterilization-of-disabled-people-in-the-united-states/ (last accessed May 2024).
88. Jenny Brown, *Birth Strike: The Hidden Fight over Women's Work* (Oakland, CA: PM Press, 2019), 127–129.
89. Brooke V. Heagerty, 'Reassessing the Guilty: The Midwives Act and the Control of English Midwives in the Early 20th Century', in *Supervision of Midwives*, ed. Mavis Kirkham (Hale, England: Books for Midwives Press, 1996), 13–27, 13. Interim measures were established which enabled the many lay midwives of the time to continue temporarily attending births. Brooke V. Heagerty,

'Willing Handmaidens of Science? The Struggle over the New Midwife in Early Twentieth-Century England', in *Reflections on Midwifery*, eds Mavis J. Kirkham and Elizabeth R. Perkins (London: Baillière Tindall, 1997), 70–95, 74.
90. Ibid., 87.
91. Ibid., 72.
92. Ibid.
93. Heagerty, 'Reassessing the Guilty', 20.
94. Ibid., 16.
95. Heagerty, 'Willing Handmaidens of Science', 81.
96. Heagerty, 'Reassessing the Guilty', 16; Heagerty, 'Willing Handmaidens of Science?', 78.
97. Heagerty, 'Reassessing the Guilty', 16.
98. Heagerty, 'Willing Handmaidens of Science?', 78.
99. Ibid., 79.
100. Heagerty, 'Reassessing the Guilty', 23.
101. Ibid., 23.
102. Heagerty, 'Willing Handmaidens of Science?', 85.
103. Evan Willis, *Medical Dominance* (Revised edition. Sydney, London and Boston, MA: Allen & Unwin, 1989).
104. Ibid., 109.
105. Ibid., 5.
106. Ibid., 6.
107. Heagerty, 'Willing Handmaidens of Science?', 188.
108. Donnison, *Midwives and Medical Men*, 177.
109. Willis, *Medical Dominance*, 107.
110. Vicente Navarro, 'Professional Dominance or Proletarianization? Neither', *The Milbank Quarterly* 66, Supplement 2: The Changing Character of the Medical Profession (1988): 57–75, 66.
111. Willis, *Medical Dominance*, 102.
112. Ibid., 111–116.
113. Ibid., 116.
114. Ibid., 93.
115. Ibid., 123.
116. Marx, *Capital, Vol. 1*, 471–72; Marx and Engels, *The German Ideology*, 33 & 44.
117. Marx and Engels, *The German Ideology*, 41.
118. Marx, *Capital, Vol.* 1, 284.
119. Mary O'Brien. *The Politics of Reproduction* (Boston, London and Henley: Routledge and Kegan Paul, 1981), 24 & 38.
120. See, for example, Maria Mies, *Patriarchy and Accumulation on a World Scale: Women in the International Division of Labour* (London: Zed Books, 2014), 51-54; Wally Seccombe, 'Marxism and Demography', *New Left Review*, I/137 (Jan/Feb 1983): 22-47, 28-29.
121. Marx, *Capital, Vol. 1*, 287.
122. Ibid., 287, fn 8. On this point see Maria Mies, *Patriarchy and Accumulation on a World Scale*, 47.
123. Marx, *Capital, Vol. 1*, 1038; original emphasis.
124. Maria Dalla Costa and Selma James, 'Women and the Subversion of the Community' in Maria Dalla Costa and Selma James, *The Power of Women and*

the Subversion of the Community (Bristol, England: Falling Wall Press Ltd., 1975), 21–56, 53 (footnote 12); original emphasis.

125. Selma James, 'Introduction', in Maria Dalla Costa and Selma James, *The Power of Women and the Subversion of the Community* (Bristol, England: Falling Wall Press Ltd., 1975), 5–20, 11.
126. Dalla Costa and James, 'Women and the Subversion of the Community', 36.
127. Leopoldina Fortunati, *The Arcane of Reproduction: Housework, Prostitution, Labor and Capital*, trans. Hilary Creek (Brooklyn, NY: Autonomedia, 1995), 71.
128. Fortunati added that, 'It could be noted here that the existence of sperm banks does not affect the argument.' Ibid., 71.
129. Ibid., 71–72.
130. Paddy Quick, 'The Class Nature of Women's Oppression', *Review of Radical Political Economics* 9, no. 3 (1977): 42–53, 46.
131. Ibid., 50–51.
132. Lise Vogel, *Marxism and the Oppression of Women* (Leiden and Boston, MA: Brill, 2013), 151.
133. Ibid., 152.
134. See, for example, Vogel, 153.
135. The argument of Paddy Quick and a range of other Marxist-feminists regarding the subjugation of women, differs considerably from that developed by Engels in *The Origin of the Family, Private Property and the State* (London: Lawrence & Wishart, 1972). In 'The Class Nature of Women's Oppression', Quick contended that Engels was correct in his 'emphasis on women's childbearing as key to understanding of the oppression of women', although for Quick such subjugation did not pertain to women as the producers of property inheritors as Engels had suggested, but to women as the producers of future workers (p. 44). For Engels, when a substantial surplus (more goods than was needed for collective survival) had historically started to be generated in pre-capitalist societies, that surplus tended to be concentrated in arenas of work (such as cattle breeding) where – due to historical and emergent divisions of labour – men predominated. In the context also of erosions in communal ownership and shifting kinship structures, men could not posthumously pass that property to their children so long as descent was determined down the maternal line (which could be proven because women gave birth to children). Engels posited that family formations thereby developed in which women came to be subordinated to a single husband as a way of facilitating female monogamy (and therefore knowledge of a child's paternity). In his own words, 'the overthrow of mother right was the *world historical defeat of the female sex*' (120). Limitations in the anthropology upon which Engels premised his work have been noted, and by the late 1970s, his work was also being called into question by a range of Marxist-feminists. (On limitations of the anthropology upon which Engel's based his argument see Eleanor Burke Leacock, 'Introduction' in Frederick Engels, *The Origin of the Family, Private Property and the State* [London: Lawrence & Wishart, 1972], 7–67, 21).
136. Lewis, *The Politics of Everybody: Feminism, Queer Theory and Marxism at the Intersection*, 182.
137. Endnotes, 'The Logic of Gender', *Endnotes* 3, September 2013, https://endnotes.org.uk/translations/endnotes-the-logic-of-gender (last accessed April 2024).

138. Ibid.; original emphasis.
139. Lewis, *Full Surrogacy Now*, 59.
140. Susan Ferguson, 'Notes on Sophie Lewis: Wombs, Value and Production', *Spectre Journal* (online), no. 1 (6 June 2020). On surrogate pregnancies and value, see also Sigrid Vertommen and Camille Barbagallo, 'The in/Visible Wombs of the Market: The Dialectics of Waged and Unwaged Reproductive Labour in the Global Surrogacy Industry', *Review of International Political Economy* 29, no. 6 (2022): 1945–1966.
141. See, for example, Marx, *Capital, Vol. 1*, 129.
142. Lewis, *Full Surrogacy Now: Feminism against Family*, 74.
143. Ferguson, 'Notes on Sophie Lewis: Wombs, Value and Production'.
144. Ibid.
145. Ibid.; original emphasis.
146. Marx, *Grundrisse*, 817.
147. Martha Gimenez, 'The Mode of Reproduction in Transition: A Marxist-Feminist Analysis of the Effects of Reproductive Technologies', *Gender & Society* 5, no. 3 (September 1991): 334–350, 341.
148. Ibid., 344; Russell makes a related argument, noting that 'the organic link between a child and a particular woman is being ruptured, and there is a separation of genetic, gestational and social parentage.' Kathryn Russell, 'A Value-theoretic Approach to Childbirth and Reproductive Engineering', *Science & Society* 58, no. 3 (1994): 287–314, 301.
149. Davis, 'Outcast Mothers and Surrogates: Racism and Reproductive Politics'.
150. Brown, *Birth Strike: The Hidden Fight over Women's Work.*
151. Nancy Fraser, 'Contradictions of Capital and Care', *New Left Review*, II, no. 100 (2016): 99–117, 114–115.
152. Ibid., 115.
153. Alys Eve Weinbaum, *The Afterlife of Reproductive Slavery: Biocapitalism and Black Feminism's Philosophy of History* (Durham, NC and London: Duke University Press, 2019).
154. See, for example, Lewis, *Full Surrogacy Now: Feminism against Family*, especially 78–80.
155. Kevin Floyd, 'Automatic Subjects: Gendered Labour and Abstract Life', *Historical Materialism* 24, no. 2 (2016): 61–86, 78–79.
156. Ibid., 78–79.
157. See, for example, Melinda Cooper, *Life as Surplus: Biotechnology and Capitalism in the Neoliberal Era* (Seattle and London: University of Washington Press, 2008); Catherine Waldby and Melinda Cooper, 'The Biopolitics of Reproduction', *Australian Feminist Studies* 23, no. 55 (1 March 2008): 57–73; Melinda Cooper and Catherine Waldby, 'From Reproductive Work to Regenerative Labour: The Female Body and the Stem Cell Industries', *Feminist Theory* 11, no. 1 (2010): 3–22.
158. Savannah Koplon, 'UAB's First Uterus Transplant Recipient Delivers Healthy Baby', *University of Alabama at Birmingham*, 24 July 2023, www.uab.edu/news/health/item/13684-uab-s-first-uterus-transplant-recipient-delivers-healthy-baby (last accessed May 2024).
159. See, for example, N. Hammond-Browning, 'UK Criteria for Uterus Transplantation: A Review', *BJOG: An International Journal of Obstetrics & Gynaecology*

126, no. 11 (2019): 1320–1326; B.P. Jones, N.J. Williams, S. Saso, M-Y Thum, I. Quiroga, J. Yazbek, S. Wilkinson, S. Ghaem-Maghami, P. Thomas and J.R. Smith, 'Uterine Transplantation in Transgender Women', *BJOG* 126, no. 2 (Jan 2019): 152–156.

160. Hammond-Browning, 'UK Criteria for Uterus Transplantation: A Review', 1322.
161. Sophie Lewis, 'Do Electric Sheep Dream of Water Babies?' *Logic Magazine*, Issue 8 (3 August 2019). https://logicmag.io/bodies/do-electric-sheep-dream-of-water-babies/ (last accessed May 2024).
162. Shulamith Firestone, *The Dialectic of Sex: The Case for Feminist Revolution* (London: The Women's Press, 1979), 14.
163. Ibid., 193; original emphasis.
164. See, for example, Nick Srnicek and Alex Williams, *Inventing the Future: Postcapitalism and a World without Work* (Verso Books, 2015); Aaron Bastani, *Fully Automated Luxury Communism* (Verso Books, 2019).
165. Lewis, *Full Surrogacy Now*, 1.
166. Silvia Federici, *Beyond the Periphery of the Skin* (PM Press, 2020), 18.
167. David Harvey, *The Limits to Capital* (London and New York, Verso, 2018. Ebook, p. 506.
168. Silvia Federici, 'Introduction', in *Birth Work as Care Work: Stories from Activist Birth Communities*, ed. Alana Apfel (Oakland, CA: PM Press, 2016), xxi–xxv, xxii.

CHAPTER 3 TECHNOLOGICAL FETISH IN THE BIRTH CHAMBER

1. Selma M. Taffel, Paul J. Placek, and Teri Liss, 'Trends in the United States Cesarean Section Rate and Reasons for the 1980–85 Rise', *American Journal of Public Health* 77, no. 8 (August 1987), 955–959; OECD Health Statistics 2019, 'Caesarean Sections. Health at a Glance 2019 – OECD Indicators', Figure 9.16, https://tinyurl.com/ujkwvfvm (last accessed May 2024).
2. NHS Digital, *NHS Maternity Statistics, England 2021–2022*. Summary report tables accessed through https://digital.nhs.uk/data-and-information/publications/statistical/nhs-maternity-statistics/2021-22 (last accessed May 2024): This information pertains to English NHS hospitals.
3. Based on 2021 data and pertaining to publicly funded birth care. Te Whatu Ora, *Report on Maternity Webtool*, New Zealand Government, https://tewhatuora.shinyapps.io/report-on-maternity-web-tool/ (last accessed May 2024).
4. Maternal Mortality 2020-2022, *National Perinatal Epidemiology Unit, MBRRACE-UK*, January 2024, www.npeu.ox.ac.uk/mbrrace-uk/data-brief/maternal-mortality-2020-2022 (last accessed June 2024); Sands and Tommy's Policy Unit, *Saving Babies' Lives 2024: A report on progress* (Sands and Tommy's Policy Unit, May 2024).
5. Sakala et al., *Listening to Mothers in California*; Lindsay Cole, Amanda LeCouteur, Rebecca Feo and Hannah Dahlen, '"Trying to Give Birth Naturally Was Out of the Question"', *Women and Birth*, 32, no. 1 (2019), e95–e101.
6. Mavis Kirkham, 'Fundamental Contradictions: The Business Model versus Midwifery Values', in *Untangling the Maternity Crisis*, eds Nadine Edwards,

Rosemary Mander and Jo Murphy-Lawless (London: Routledge, 2018), 75–83, 78.

7. According to The International Federation of Gynecology and Obstetrics, 'Worldwide there is an alarming increase in caesarean section (CS) rates. The medical profession on its own cannot reverse this trend.' Gerard H. A. Visser, Diogo Ayres-de-Campos, Eytan R. Barnea, Luc de Bernis, Gian Carlo Di Renzo, Maria Fernanda Escobar Vidarte, Isabel Lloyd, Anwar H. Nassar, Wanda Nicholson, P. K. Shah, William Stones, Luming Sun, Gerhard B. Theron and Salimah Walani, 'FIGO Position Paper: How to Stop the Caesarean Section Epidemic', *The Lancet* 392, no. 10155 (October 2018): 1286–1287, 1286.
8. Marx, *Grundrisse*, 693.
9. Robert Angus Buchanan, 'History of Technology', *Encyclopedia Britannica*, 4 March 2024, www.britannica.com/technology/history-of-technology (last accessed May 2024).
10. There is a recorded case of a woman surviving a caesarean in 1500 in Switzerland. Donald Todman, 'A History of Caesarean Section: From Ancient World to the Modern Era: A History of Caesarean Section', *Australian and New Zealand Journal of Obstetrics and Gynaecology* 47, no. 5 (14 September 2007): 357–361, 358. In the Kingdom of Bunyoro-Kitara, Africa, practices of caesarean section which saved both mother and child date from before the 1880s. J. N. P. Davies, 'The Development of "Scientific" Medicine in the African Kingdom of Bunyoro-Kitaram', *Medical History* 3, no. 1 (January 1957): 47–57.
11. Hilary Marland, 'The "Burgerlijke" Midwife: The Stadsvroedvrouw of Eighteenth-Century Holland', in *The Art of Midwifery: Early Modern Midwives in Europe*, ed. Hilary Marland (London & New York: Routledge, 1993), 193–213, 193; R. E. Evenden, cited in Maria Kontoyannis and Christos Katsetos, 'Midwives in Early Modern Europe (1400–1800)', *Health Science Journal* 5, no. 1 (2011), 31–36, 33.
12. Donnison, *Midwives and Medical Men*, 34.
13. Peter M. Dunn, 'The Chamberlen Family (1560–1728) and Obstetric Forceps', *Archives of Disease in Childhood – Fetal and Neonatal Edition* 81, no. 3 (1999), F232–234.
14. Harvey Graham, *Eternal Eve* (London: William Heinemann – Medical Books Ltd, 1950), 188.
15. James Drife, 'The Start of Life: A History of Obstetrics', *Postgraduate Medical Journal* 78, no. 919 (2002): 311–315, 312.
16. Donnison, *Midwives and Medical Men*, 34.
17. Adrian Wilson, 'Midwifery in the "Medical Marketplace"' in *Medicine and the Market in England and its Colonies, c. 1450–c. 1850*, eds Mark S. R. Jenner and Patrick Wallis (London: Palgrave Macmillan, 2007), 153–174, 167.
18. Loudon, 'Maternal Mortality in the Past and Its Relevance to Developing Countries Today', 243S.
19. Joseph B. DeLee, 'The Prophylactic Forceps Operation', *American Journal of Obstetrics and Gynecology* 1 (1920): 34–44.
20. Ibid., 44.
21. Joseph B. DeLee, 'Progress toward Ideal Obstetrics', *The American Journal of Obstetrics and Diseases of Women and Children (1869–1919)* 73, no. 3 (1916): 407–415, 407.

22. Danielle Thompson, 'Midwives and Pregnant Women of Color: Why We Need to Understand Intersectional Changes in Midwifery to Reclaim Home Birth', *Columbia Journal of Race & Law* 6 (2016): 27–46, 28–30.
23. Keisha Goode and Barbara Katz Rothman, 'African-American Midwifery, a History and a Lament', *The American Journal of Economics and Sociology* 76, no. 1 (2017): 65–94, 72.
24. Harriet A. Washington, *Medical Apartheid* (New York: Harlem Moon, Broadway Books, 2008), 66.
25. Vanessa Northington Gamble, featuring in Shankar Vedantam and Maggie Penman, 'Remembering Anarcha, Lucy, and Betsey: The Mothers of Modern Gynecology', *The Hidden Brain*, Podcast, National Public Radio. 16 February 2016. www.npr.org/2016/02/16/466942135/remembering-anarcha-lucy-and-betsey-the-mothers-of-modern-gynecology (last accessed May 2024).
26. Vedantam and Penman, 'Remembering Anarcha, Lucy, and Betsey'.
27. Judith Walzer Leavitt, 'Birthing and Anaesthesia: The Debate over Twilight Sleep', *Signs* 6, no. 1 (1980): 147–164.
28. Doris C. Gordon and Francis Bennett, *Gentlemen of the Jury* (New Plymonth, NZ: Thomas Avery & Sons Limited, 1937), 17, 18.
29. Doris Gordon, *Backblocks Baby-Doctor: An Autobiography by Doris Gordon* (London: Faber & Faber Limited, 1955), 158, 159.
30. Jane Stojanovic, 'Midwifery in New Zealand 1904–1971', *Contemporary Nurse* 30, no. 2 (1 October 2008): 156–167, 159.
31. Barbara Katz Rothman, *In Labor: Women and Power in the Birthplace* (New York and London: W. W. Norton & Company, 1982), 34.
32. Robbie E. Davis-Floyd, 'The Technological Model of Birth', *The Journal of American Folklore* 100, no. 398 (1987): 479–495; Davis-Floyd, 'The Technocratic and Holistic Models of Birth Compared', *Special Delivery*, Winter (1991): 10; Davis-Floyd, 'The Technocratic, Humanistic, and Holistic Paradigms of Childbirth', *International Journal of Gynecology & Obstetrics* 75, no. S1 (2001): S5–23. For discussion of Davis-Floyd's renaming of the model from 'technological' to 'technocratic', see Davis-Floyd, 'The Technocratic Body: American Childbirth as Cultural Expression', *Social Science & Medicine* 38, no. 8 (1994): 1125–1140, 1139–1140 (fn 2).
33. Davis-Floyd, 'The Technocratic, Humanistic, and Holistic Paradigms of Childbirth', S9.
34. See, for example, Davis-Floyd, 'The Technocratic Body: American Childbirth as Cultural Expression'.
35. Louise Marie Roth. *The Business of Birth: Malpractice and Maternity Care in the United States* (New York: New York University Press, 2021), 28.
36. David Harvey, 'The Fetish of Technology: Causes and Consequences', *Macalester International* 13, article 7 (2003): 3–30, 3.
37. Harvey, 'The Fetish of Technology', 3.
38. For Marx on the fetishism of the commodity, see Marx, *Capital, Vol. 1*, 164–177.
39. Slavoj Žižek, *The Sublime Object of Ideology* (London and New York: Verso, 1989), 50.
40. Harvey, 'The Fetish of Technology'.
41. Ibid., 6.
42. Ibid., 7.

43. Ibid., 7.
44. Marx, *Grundrisse*, 692–693.
45. Ibid., 693.
46. Marx, *Capital, Vol. 1*, 342.
47. Ibid., 644.
48. Ibid., 644.
49. Susan Ferguson, *Women and Work: Feminism, Labour and Social Reproduction* (London: Pluto Press, 2020), 126.
50. Denis Walsh, 'Subverting the Assembly-Line: Childbirth in a Free-Standing Birth Centre', *Social Science & Medicine* 62, no. 6 (2006): 1330–1340, 1332.
51. Kieran O'Driscoll, John M. Stronge, and Maurice Minogue. 'Active Management of Labour', *British Medical Journal* 3, no. 21 (July 1973): 135–137, 135.
52. Ibid., 135.
53. Ibid., 137.
54. Ibid., 136.
55. Karyn J. Kaufman, 'Effective Control or Effective Care', *Birth* 20, no. 3 (1993): 156–158, 157.
56. See, for example, William Fraser, 'Methodologic Issues in Assessing the Active Management of Labor', *Birth* 20, no. 3 (1993): 155–156, 156.
57. Niles Newton, cited in Michel Odent, *The Scientification of Love* (London: Free Association Books, 1999), 10.
58. Michel Odent, *Childbirth in the Age of Plastics* (London: Pinter & Martin Ltd., 2011): 4–7.
59. Walsh, 'Subverting the Assembly-Line', 1332–1333.
60. Kieran O'Driscoll and Declan Meagher with Peter Boylan, *Active Management of Labor: The Dublin Experience*, 3rd edition (London: Mosby, 1993), 113.
61. Ibid., 114.
62. On Taylorism in birth care see Walsh, 'Subverting the Assembly-Line', 1333–1334.
63. O'Driscoll, Meagher and Boylan, *Active Management of Labor: The Dublin Experience*, 96–103.
64. Ibid., 115.
65. Perkins, *The Medical Delivery Business*, 155.
66. Harry Braverman, *Labor and Monopoly Capital: The Degradation of Work in the Twentieth Century*, 25th Anniversary Edition, Digital (New York: Monthly Review Press, 1998), 94.
67. Ibid., 103.
68. Ibid., 140.
69. See, for example, Tony Farmer, *Holles Street 1894–1994* (Dublin: A.A. Farmar, 1994), 155–157.
70. O'Driscoll, Meagher and Boylan, *Active Management of Labor: The Dublin Experience*, 115.
71. Perkins, *Medical Delivery Business*, 148–49.
72. O'Driscoll, Meagher and Boylan, *Active Management of Labor: The Dublin Experience*, 114.
73. The Editor, 'The Essential Midwife', *AIMS – Association for Improvements in the Maternity Services* [from *Aims Journal* 10, no. 2 (1998)] www.aims.org.uk/journal/item/the-essential-midwife (last accessed May 2024).

74. See, for example, Meghan A. Bohren, G. Justus Hofmeyr, Carol Sakala, Rieko K. Fukuzawa and Anna Cuthbert, 'Continuous Support for Women During Childbirth', *Cochrane Database of Systematic Reviews*, 7, 7 (2017): CD003766.
75. Kieran O'Driscoll, Michael Foley and Dermot MacDonald, 'Active Management of Labor as an Alternative to Cesarean Section for Dystocia', *Obstetrics & Gynecology* 63, no. 4 (1984): 485–490.
76. J. G. Thornton and R. J. Lilford, 'Active Management of Labour: Current Knowledge and Research Issues', *BMJ* 309, no. 6951 (6 August 1994): 366–369, 368.
77. J. G. Thornton, 'Active Management of Labour', *BMJ* 313, no. 7054 (17 August 1996): 378.
78. Heather C. Brown, Shantini Paranjothy, Therese Dowswell and Jane Thomas, 'Package of Care for Active Management in Labour for Reducing Caesarean Section Rates in Low-Risk Women', *Cochrane Database of Systematic Reviews*, no. 9 (2013), 2.
79. Sheryl Burt Ruzek, 'Defining Reducible Risk: Social Dimensions of Assessing Birth Technologies', *Human Nature* 4, no. 4 (1993): 383–408, 401.
80. Ibid., 401.
81. Perkins, *Medical Delivery Business*, 138.
82. Data from 'RCM Members Experience Survey' conducted in August 2021, reported in Royal College of Midwives, 'RCM Warns of Midwife Exodus as Maternity Staffing Crisis Grows', *Royal College of Midwives*, 4 October 2021, www.rcm.org.uk/media-releases/2021/september/rcm-warns-of-midwife-exodus-as-maternity-staffing-crisis-grows/ (last accessed May 2024).
83. Black Mamas Matter Alliance (lead author Sunshine Muse, contributing authors Elizabeth Dawes Gay, Angela Doyinsola Aina, Carmen Green, Joia Crear-Perry, Jessica Roach, Haguerenesh Tesfa, Kay Matthews and Tanay L. Harris), *Setting the Standard for Holistic Care of and for Black Women* (Atlanta, GA: Black Mamas Matter Alliance, April 2018), 23.
84. Cornel M. Angolile, Baraka L. Max, Justice Mushemba and Harold L. Mashauri, 'Global Increased Cesarean Section Rates and Public Health Implications: A Call to Action', *Health Science Reports* 6, no. 5 (18 May 2023), e1274.
85. World Health Organization, *WHO Statement on Caesarean Section Rates* (Geneva: World Health Organization, 2015).
86. World Health Organization, *WHO Recommendations: Non-Clinical Interventions to Reduce Unnecessary Caesarean Sections* (Geneva: World Health Organization, 2018), 49.
87. Robert Pearl, 'US Healthcare: A Conglomerate of Monopolies', *Forbes*, 16 January 2023, https://tinyurl.com/yv66zva4 (last accessed May 2024).
88. Walsh, 'Subverting the Assembly-Line', 1333.
89. O'Driscoll, Meagher and Boylan, *Active Management of Labor: The Dublin Experience*, 113.
90. Private-sector doctor (research participant) quoted in Alison Peel, Abhishek Bhartia, Neil Spicer and Meenakshi Gautham, '"If I Do 10–15 Normal Deliveries in a Month I Hardly Ever Sleep at Home." A Qualitative Study of Health Providers' Reasons for High Rates of Caesarean Deliveries in Private Sector Maternity Care in Delhi, India', *BMC Pregnancy and Childbirth* 18, no. 470 (2018): 4.

91. Jonah Bardos, Holly Loudon, Patricia Rekawek, Frederick Friedman, Michael Brodman and Nathan S. Fox, 'The Association Between Solo Versus Group Obstetrical Practice Model and Delivery Outcomes', *American Journal of Perinatology* 36, no. 9 (2019): 907–910.
92. World Health Organization. *WHO Recommendations: Non-Clinical Interventions to Reduce Unnecessary Caesarean Sections*, 11
93. Melissa G. Rosenstein, Malini Nijagal, Sanae Nakagawa, Steven E. Gregorich and Miriam Kuppermann, 'The Association of Expanded Access to a Collaborative Midwifery and Laborist Model With Cesarean Delivery Rates', *Obstetrics and Gynecology* 126, no. 4 (October 2015): 716–723, 722.
94. C. Edward Wells, 'A Transition in Obstetrics', *American Medical Association Journal of Ethics* (*Virtual Mentor*) 10, no. 12 (2008): 823–828, 824.
95. Theresa Morris, Kelly McNamara and Christine H. Morton, 'Hospital-Ownership Status and Cesareans in the United States: The Effect of for-Profit Hospitals', *Birth* 44, no. 4 (2017): 325–330.
96. Ibid., 327.
97. See, for example, Marx, *Capital, Vol. 1*, 777–778; Karl Marx, *Capital, Vol. 3*, trans. David Fernbach (Harmondsworth: Penguin Books, 1981), Part Five.
98. Costas Lapavitsas, 'The Financialization of Capitalism: "Profiting without Producing"', *City* 17, no. 6 (2013): 792–805.
99. Paul M. Sweezy, 'The Triumph of Financial Capital', *Monthly Review* 46, no. 2 (1994): 1–11.
100. Arnold S. Relman, 'The New Medical-Industrial Complex', *New England Journal of Medicine* (23 October 1980).
101. Morris et al., 'Hospital-Ownership Status and Cesareans in the United States: The Effect of for-Profit Hospitals', 328.
102. Joseph Dov Bruch, Victor Roy and Colleen M. Grogan, 'The Financialization of Health in the United States', *Medicine and Society*, 11 January 2024, 178–182, 178.
103. Ibid., 181.
104. World Health Organization, *WHO Recommendations: Non-Clinical Interventions to Reduce Unnecessary Caesarean Sections*, 11.
105. See, for example, Ilir Hoxha, Lamprini Syrogiannouli, Medina Braha, David C. Goodman, Bruno R. da Costa and Peter Jüni, 'Caesarean Sections and Private Insurance: Systematic Review and Meta-Analysis', *BMJ Open* 7, no. 7 (2017): e016600: 4, 8.
106. Philip Zwecker, Laurent Azoulay and Haim A. Abenhaim, 'Effect of Fear of Litigation on Obstetric Care: A Nationwide Analysis on Obstetric Practice', *American Journal of Perinatology* 28, no. 4 (2011): 277–284.
107. Steven M. Rock, 'Malpractice Premiums and Primary Caesarean Section Rates in New York and Illinois', *Public Health Reports* 103, no. 5 (1988): 459–463, 460.
108. Carol Sakala, Y. Tony Yang and Maureen P. Corry, *Maternity Care and Liability: Pressing Problems, Substantive Solutions* (New York: Childbirth Connection, January 2013), 24. https://nationalpartnership.org/wp-content/uploads/2023/02/maternity-care-and-liability-report.pdf (last accessed May 2024).
109. Ibid., 18.

110. See, for example, Tricia Anderson, 'Insurance and British Midwifery: The End of Independent Midwifery in the UK', *Midwifery Today* (Summer 2007): 55–56.
111. Jacqui Tomkins in KGH, 'Have We Lost Independent Midwives Forever?', KGH, 2021, www.youtube.com/watch?v=Lx2UBYrJBrw (last accessed May 2024): 56:50.
112. Milena Canil, 'Australia's Insurance Crisis and the Inequitable Treatment of Self-employed Midwives', *Australia and New Zealand Health Policy* 5, no. 6 (29 May 2008).
113. Slavoj Žižek describes a fetish, in the work of Freud, as concealing 'the lack ... around which the symbolic network is articulated'. *The Sublime Object of Ideology* (London and New York: Verso), 50.
114. Jane Evans, Personal Communication, March 2003.
115. Murray W. Enkin, Sholom Glouberman, Philip Groff, Alejandro R. Jadad and Anita Stern, 'Beyond Evidence: The Complexity of Maternity Care', *Birth* 33, no. 4 (2006): 265–269, 265.
116. Miranda Page and Rosemary Mander, 'Intrapartum Uncertainty: A Feature of Normal Birth, as Experienced by Midwives in Scotland', *Midwifery* 30, no. 1 (2014): 28–35, 31; Neel Shah, 'The Surprising Factor Behind a Spike in C-Sections', interview by Noah Leavitt, *Harvard Chan: This Week in Health*, 27 July 2017, https://www.hsph.harvard.edu/news/multimedia-article/csections-delivery-risk-podcast/ (last accessed August 2024).
117. Claire L. Wendland, 'The Vanishing Mother: Cesarean Section and "Evidence-Based Obstetrics"', *Medical Anthropology Quarterly* 21, no. 2 (2007): 218–233, 218. Sociologist Wendy Simonds also writes that from a midwifery perspective 'The cultural portrayal of birth, abetted by obstetrics, depicts it as risky and fearful, and interventions as protecting women against the overwhelming pain and providing control over the uncertainty.' Simonds, 'Birth Matters: Practicing Midwifery', in *Laboring On: Birth In Transition in the United States*, eds Wendy Simonds, Barbara Katz Rothman and Bari Meltzer Norman(New York and Oxford: Routledge, 2007): 155–206, 205.
118. Robbie E. Davis-Floyd, 'The Role of Obstetric Rituals in the Resolution of Cultural Anomaly', *Social Science of Medicine* 31, no. 2 (1990): 175–189, 181.
119. Shah, 'The Surprising Factor Behind a Spike in C-Sections', interview. With regards to my use of this quotation, I value the work of Neel Shah, and consider the fact that he is able to articulate such a dilemma as testimony to his insights into the field.
120. Ibid.
121. Ibid.
122. Ibid.
123. Christina Brigance, Ripley Lucas, Erin Jones, Ann Davis, Motoko Oinuma, Kate Mishkin and Zsakeba Henderson, *Nowhere to Go: Maternity Care Deserts Across the U.S.*, March of Dimes Report No.3. (2022), www.marchofdimes.org/sites/default/files/2022-10/2022_Maternity_Care_Report.pdf (last accessed May 2024).
124. Ibid.
125. United States Government Accountability Office, *Rural Hospital Closures: Affected Residents had Reduced Access to Healthcare Services* (Report to the Ranking Member, Committee on Homeland Security and Governmental

Affairs, United States Senate, December 2020), 20. www.gao.gov/assets/gao-21-93.pdf (last accessed May 2024).

126. Miller, Abalos, Chamillard et al., 'Beyond Too Little, Too Late and Too Much, Too Soon'.
127. Mason Boycott-Owen and Laura Donnelly, 'Women in Labour are Being Denied Epidurals by the NHS, Amid Concern Over "Cult of Natural Childbirth"', *The Telegraph*, 24 January 2020, https://tinyurl.com/3v5mrcaf (last accessed May 2024); Amelia Hill, '"I Asked Three Times for an Epidural": Why Are Women Being Denied Pain Relief During Childbirth?' *The Guardian*, 4 March 2020, https://tinyurl.com/2ar2n437 (last accessed May 2024).
128. David Bogod, 'Epidural Denial. Thoughts from the Frontline', *Royal College of Anaesthetists*, 29 January 2020, https://rcoa.ac.uk/blog/epidural-denial-thoughts-frontline (last accessed May 2024).
129. Hill, '"I Asked Three Times for an Epidural"'.
130. Marsden Wagner, *Pursuing the Birth Machine: The Search for Appropriate Birth Technology* (Camperdown, Australia: ACE Graphics, 1994).
131. Fredric Jameson, 'An American Utopia', in *An American Utopia: Dual Power and the Universal Army*, ed. Slavoj Žižek (London and New York: Verso, 2016): 1–96, 49.
132. Wagner, *Pursuing the Birth Machine: The Search for Appropriate Birth Technology*, 20.
133. Fredric Jameson, *Representing Capital: A Reading of Volume 1* (Verso, 2014, ebook edition), Introduction, paragraph 12.
134. Ibid.

CHAPTER 4 SUBSUMED BY RISK

1. Williamson also makes this point specifically in relation to childbirth in Brazil. K. Eliza Williamson and Etsuko Matsuoka, 'Comparing Childbirth in Brazil and Japan: Social Hierarchies, Cultural Values, and the Meaning of Place', in *In Birth in Eight Cultures*, eds Robbie Davis-Floyd and Melissa Cheyney (Long Grove, IL: Waveland Press Inc., 2019), 89–128, 99.
2. Barbara Katz Rothman, 'Editorial: Pregnancy, Birth and Risk – An Introduction', *Health, Risk & Society* 16, no. 1 (2 January 2014): 1–6, 1.
3. Beck, *Risk Society: Towards a New Modernity* (London: SAGE Publications, Inc., 1992).
4. Ibid., 155.
5. Ulrich Beck, 'This Free-market Farce Shows How Badly We Need the State', *The Guardian*, 10 April 2008, www.theguardian.com/business/2008/apr/10/creditcrunch.economics (last accessed May 2024).
6. Marx, *Capital, Volume 1*, 1019–38.
7. Peter L. Bernstein, *Against the Gods: The Remarkable Story of Risk* (New York: John Wiley & Sons, Inc., electronic edition, 1998), 13.
8. Ibid.
9. Karl Marx, *Theories of Surplus-Value [Vol. IV of Capital]* (Progress Publishers, Mark-up by Hans G. Ehrar) [The Absurdity of Speaking of Wages as an Advance by the Capitalist to the Labourer. Bourgeois Competition of Profit as Reward

for Risk] www.marxists.org/archive/marx/works/1863/theories-surplus-value/ch06.htm#s3a (last accessed May 2024).
10. Ibid.
11. Bernstein, *Against the Gods*, 14.
12. Ibid., 107.
13. Lauren Fordyce and Amínata Maraesa, 'Introduction: The Development of Discourses Surrounding Reproductive Risks', in *Risk, Reproduction, and Narratives of Experience*, eds Lauren Fordyce and Amínata Maraesa (Nashville, TN: Vanderbilt University Press, 2012), 1–13, 1.
14. Elizabeth Cartwright and Jan Thomas, 'Constructing Risk: Maternity Care, Law, and Malpractice', in *Birth by Design: Pregnancy, Maternity Care, and Midwifery in North America and Europe*, eds Raymond De Vries, Cecilia Benoit, Edwin R. Teijlingen and Sirpa Wrede (New York and London: Routledge, 2001), 218–28, 218.
15. Julia Allison, *Midwifery from the Tudors to the 21st Century* (London and New York: Routledge, 2021), 44.
16. Elizabeth Nihell, *A Treatise on the Art of Midwifery. Setting Forth Various Abuses Therein, Especially as to the Practice with Instruments: The Whole Serving to Put All Rational Inquirers in a Fair Way of Very Safely Forming Their Own Judgment upon the Question; Which It Is Best to Employ, in Cases of Pregnancy and Lying-in, a Man-Midwife; or, a Midwife* (London: Printed for A. Morley, 1760), 386.
17. Ibid., 78.
18. William Smellie, *A Treatise on the Theory and Practice of Midwifery (Vol. 1)* (London: D. Wilson and T. Durham, 1766, Fifth edition corrected, Ebook), 247.
19. Figures based upon 2011 data. Jane Sandall, Trevor Murrells, Miranda Dodwell, Rod Gibson, Susan Bewley, Kirstie Coxon, Debra Bick, Graham Cookson, Cathy Warwick and Diana Hamilton-Fairley, 'The Efficient Use of the Maternity Workforce and the Implications for Safety and Quality in Maternity Care: A Population-Based, Cross-Sectional Study', *Health Services and Delivery Research* 2, no. 38 (October 2014): 35, 73.
20. Marianne P. Amelink-Verburg and Simone E. Buitendijk, 'Pregnancy and Labour in the Dutch Maternity Care System: What Is Normal? The Role Division Between Midwives and Obstetricians', *Journal of Midwifery & Women's Health* 55, no. 3 (1 May 2010): 216–25, 220.
21. Eugene Declercq and Neel Shah, 'Maternal Deaths Represent the Canary in the Coal Mine for Women's Health', *STAT*, 22 August 2018, www.statnews.com/2018/08/22/maternal-deaths-women-health/ (last accessed May 2024).
22. Mandie Scamell and Andy Alaszewski, Fateful Moments and the Categorisation of Risk: Midwifery Practice and the Ever-Narrowing Window of Normality During Childbirth', *Health, Risk & Society* 14, no. 2 (2012): 207–221, 219.
23. Marx, *Capital, Vol. 1*, 1019–23.
24. Ibid., 1025.
25. Ibid., 432.
26. Ibid., 1036.
27. Toni Negri, 'Twenty Theses on Marx: Interpretation of the Class Situation Today', in *Marxism Beyond Marxism*, eds Saree Makdisi, Cesare Casarino and Rebecca E. Karl (New York and London: Routledge, 1996), 149–80, 149.

28. Silvia Federici, 'Notes on Gender in Marx's Capital', *Continental Thought and Theory* 1, no. 4 (2017): 19–37, 30.
29. Ibid., 30.
30. Jacques Camatte, *Capital and Community: The Results of the Immediate Process of Production and the Economic Work of Marx*, trans. David Brown (trans. originally published London: Unpopular Books, 1988; transcription, mark-up and minor editing, Rob Lucas, 2006), 72. www.marxists.org/archive/camatte/capcom/camatte-capcom.pdf (last accessed May 2024). This quotation from Camatte is also cited in Endnotes, 'The History of Subsumption', *Endnotes* 2 (April 2010), https://endnotes.org.uk/articles/the-history-of-subsumption (last accessed May 2024).
31. I take this point from Camatte, *Capital and Community*, 72.
32. Endnotes, 'The History of Subsumption'.
33. Ibid.
34. Ferguson, *Women and Work: Feminism, Labour and Social Reproduction*, 126.
35. Ernest Mandel, *Late Capitalism.*, trans. Joris De Bres (London: NLB, 1975), 121.
36. Nancy Fraser, 'Contradictions of Capital and Care', *New Left Review* II, no. 100 (2016): 99–117, 109.
37. Ibid., 100.
38. Ibid., 109–110.
39. On shifts in epidemiology see Neil Pearce, 'Traditional Epidemiology, Modern Epidemiology, and Public Health', *American Journal of Public Health* 86, no. 5 (1996): 678–683; Lorna Weir, *Pregnancy, Risk and Biopolitics: On the Threshold of the Living Subject* (London and New York: Routledge, 2006), 58.
40. Syed S. Mahmood, Daniel Levy, Ramachandran S. Vasan and Thomas J. Wang, 'The Framingham Heart Study and the Epidemiology of Cardiovascular Disease: A Historical Perspective', *Lancet* 383, no. 9921 (2014): 999–1008. For discussion of initial intentions regarding the study, see Mervyn Susser, 'Epidemiology in the United States after World War II: The Evolution of Technique', *Epidemiologic Reviews* 7, no. 1 (1985): 147–177, 157.
41. W. C. W. Nixon, 'Foreward', in Neville R. Butler and Dennis F. Bonham, *Perinatal Mortality: The First Report of the 1958 British Perinatal Mortality Survey under the Auspices of The National Birthday Trust Fund* (Edinburgh and London: E. & S. Livingstone Ltd., 1963), iv.
42. Neville R. Butler and Dennis F. Bonham, *Perinatal Mortality: The First Report of the 1958 British Perinatal Mortality Survey under the Auspices of The National Birthday Trust Fund* (Edinburgh & London: E. & S. Livingstone Ltd., 1963), 2–3.
43. Ibid., 34, 36.
44. Ibid., 60.
45. The Editorial Team, 'The Effects of Smoking in Pregnancy', in *Perinatal Problems: The Second Report of the 1958 British Perinatal Mortality Survey under the auspieces of The National Birthday Trust Fund*, eds Neville R. Butler and Eva D. Alberman (Edinburgh and London: E. & S. Livingstone Ltd. 1969), 72–84.
46. Weir, *Pregnancy, Risk and Biopolitics*, 59.
47. Ibid., 60.

48. Northern Regional Health Authority Coordinating Group, 'Perinatal Mortality: A Continuing Collaborative Regional Survey', *British Medical Journal (Clin. Res. Ed.)* 288 (1984): 1717–1720.
49. See, for example, Eugene Declercq, 'The Absolute Power of Relative Risk in Debates on Repeat Cesareans and Home Birth in the United States', *Journal of Clinical Ethics* 24, no. 3 (2013): 215–224.
50. Butler and Bonham, *Perinatal Mortality: The First Report of the 1958 British Perinatal Mortality Survey*, 38.
51. Weir, *Pregnancy, Risk and Biopolitics*, 60.
52. Diogo Ayres-de-Campos, 'Electronic Fetal Monitoring or Cardiotocography, 50 Years Later: What's in a Name?', *American Journal of Obstetrics and Gynecology* 218, no. 6 (2018): 545–546.
53. Malcolm Nicolson and John E. E. Fleming, *Imaging and Imagining the Fetus: The Development of Obstetric Ultrasound* (Baltimore, MD: Johns Hopkins University Press, 2013), 171.
54. Ibid., 232.
55. See, for example, National Screening Unit, *Antenatal Screening for Down Syndrome and Other Conditions: 2018 Monitoring Report* (Wellington: National Screening Unit, New Zealand, 2021), 8.
56. See, for example, ibid., 11.
57. 'Risks, Amniocentesis', *National Health Service,* (page last reviewed 12 October 2022), https://www.nhs.uk/conditions/amniocentesis/risks/ (last accessed July 2024).
58. For information on NIPT, see Janet Crofts, 'Non-Invasive Prenatal Testing (NIPT)', *Healthify*, page last updated 3 August 2022, https://healthify.nz/health-a-z/n/non-invasive-prenatal-testing-nipt/ (last accessed May 2024).
59. Ian Donald, quoted in Nicolson and Fleming, *Imaging and Imagining the Fetus*, 80.
60. Tim Jancelewicz and Michael R. Harrison, 'A History of Fetal Surgery', *Clinics in Perinatology* 36, no. 2 (2009): 227–236, 231.
61. Carol Hindley, Sophie Wren Hinsliff and Ann M. Thomson, 'English Midwives' Views and Experiences of Intrapartum Fetal Heart Rate Monitoring in Women at Low Obstetric Risk: Conflicts and Compromises', *Journal of Midwifery & Women's Health* 51, no. 5 (2006): 354–360.
62. Zarko Alfirevic, Gillian M. L. Gyte, Anna Cuthbert and Declan Devane, 'Continuous Cardiotocography (CTG) as a Form of Electronic Fetal Monitoring (EFM) for Fetal Assessment during Labour (Review)', *Cochrane Database of Systematic Reviews*, no. 2 (2017), Art No. CD006066; Lisa Heelan-Fancher, Ling Shi, Yuqing Zhang, Yurun Cai, Ampicha Nawai and Suzanne Leveille, 'Impact of Continuous Electronic Fetal Monitoring on Birth Outcomes in Low-Risk Pregnancies', *Birth* 46, no. 2 (2019): 311–317; Kirsten A. Small, Mary Sidebotham, Jennifer Fenwick and Jenny Gamble, 'Intrapartum Cardiotocograph Monitoring and Perinatal Outcomes for Women at Risk: Literature Review', *Women and Birth* 33, no. 5 (September 2020): 411–418.
63. Small et al., 'Intrapartum Cardiotocograph Monitoring and Perinatal Outcomes for Women at Risk': 411–418.
64. Ibid., 417.

65. Research participant, quoted in Maria Galea, Nicole Borg Cunen and Rita Pace Parascandalo, 'Midwives' Perspective on the Use of Intermittent Fetal Auscultation and Continuous Cardiotocography During Labour', *MIDIRS Midwifery Digest* 33, no. 3 (2023): 259–266, 262.
66. Hindley, Hinsliff and Thomson, 'English Midwives' Views and Experiences of Intrapartum Fetal Heart Rate Monitoring in Women at Low Obstetric Risk: 354–360.
67. See, for example, Alfirevic et al., 'Continuous Cardiotocography (CTG) as a Form of Electronic Fetal Monitoring (EFM) for Fetal Assessment during Labour (Review)', 7, 8.
68. This argument draws upon the work of Kirsten Small, 'Overdiagnosis and CTG monitoring', *Birth Small Talk*, 6 December 2023, https://birthsmalltalk.com/2023/12/06/overdiagnosis-and-ctg-monitoring/ (last accessed May 2024).
69. Soo Downe and Christine McCourt, 'From Being to Becoming: Reconstructing Childbirth Knowledges', in *Normal Childbirth: Evidence and Debate*, ed. Soo Downe (Edinburgh: Churchill Livingstone, Elsevier, 2008), 3–27, 10.
70. Ibid., 10.
71. Mark Richard Greene, 'Insurance – Historical Development of Insurance', *Encyclopedia Britannica*, 16 May 2024, www.britannica.com/money/insurance/Historical-development-of-insurance (last accessed May 2024).
72. A. Honeycutt, L. Dunlap, H. Chen, G. al Homsi, S. Grosse and D. Schendel, 'Economic Costs Associated with Mental Retardation, Cerebral Palsy, Hearing Loss, and Vision Impairment', *Morbidity and Mortality Weekly Report* 53, no. 3 (30 January 2004): 57–59.
73. Michael Oliver, *The Politics of Disablement* (London: MacMillan Press, 1990), 11.
74. Andrew Dickson, 'The 'No Fault' Fallacy: Looking Back at our 18 Months of ACC Hell', *The Spinoff*, 29 September 2018, https://thespinoff.co.nz/parenting/29-09-2018/the-no-fault-fallacy-looking-back-at-our-18-months-of-acc-hell?amp= (last accessed May 2024).
75. Carol Sakala, Y. Tony Yang and Maureen P. Corry, 'Maternity Care and Liability: Pressing Problems, Substantive Solutions', *Women's Health Issues* 23, no. 1 (2013): e7–e13, e8, e11.
76. Kim Price, 'Towards a History of Medical Negligence', *The Lancet* 375, no.9710 (2010): 192–193, 192.
77. Richard E. Anderson, 'Billions for Defense: The Pervasive Nature of Defensive Medicine', *Archives of Internal Medicine* 159, no. 20 (1999): 2399–2402, 2399.
78. Midwife research participant Natalie (pseudonym), quoted in Z. Spendlove, 'Risk and Boundary Work in Contemporary Maternity Care: Tensions and Consequences', *Health, Risk & Society* 20, no.1–2 (2018): 23-40, 32.
79. Midwife research participant Sue (pseudonym) quoted in ibid., 32.
80. Health and Social Care Committee, *The Safety of Maternity Services in England*, UK Parliament, 6 July 2021 (Section: Ending the Blame Culture and Establishing a Learning Culture), https://publications.parliament.uk/pa/cm5802/cmselect/cmhealth/19/1902.htm (last accessed May 2024); Edd Church, 'NMC to Investigate Claims It Hosts "Culture of Fear"', *Nursing Times*, 26 September 2023, www.nursingtimes.net/news/professional-regulation/

nmc-to-investigate-claims-it-hosts-culture-of-fear-26-09-2023/ (last accessed May 2024).

81. See, for example, Marsden Wagner, 'A Global Witch-hunt', *The Lancet* 346, no. 8981 (1995): 1020–1022; Hannah Dahlen and Jo Hunter, 'The Modern-day Witch Hunt' in *Birthing Outside the System: The Canary in the Coal Mine*, eds Hannah Dahlen, Bashi Kumar-Hazard and Virginia Schmied (Routledge, 2020): 236–255.
82. Dahlen and Hunter, 'The Modern-day Witch Hunt', 238.
83. Jacqueline Wier 'Protecting the Public: An Investigation of Midwives' Perceptions of Regulation and the Regulator', *Midwifery* 52 (2017): 57–63.
84. Research participated, quoted in Ruth Surtees, '"Everybody expects the perfect baby … and perfect labour … and so you have to protect yourself": Discourses of Defence in Midwifery Practice in Aotearoa/New Zealand', *Nursing Inquiry* 17, no. 1 (2010): 82–92, 85.
85. See, for example, Ilpo Helén, 'Technics Over Life: Risk, Ethics and the Existential Condition in High-Tech Antenatal Care', *Economy and Society* 33, no. 1 (2004): 28–51; Alphia Possamai-Inesedy, 'Confining Risk: Choice and Responsibility in Childbirth in a Risk Society', *Health Sociology Review* 15, no. 4 (1 October 2006): 406–14.
86. Slavoj Žižek, 'Risk Society and Its Discontents', *Historical Materialism* 2, no. 1 (1998): 143–64, 150–151.
87. Ibid., 151.
88. Jo Murphy-Lawless, *Reading Birth and Death: A History of Obstetric Thinking* (Cork: Cork University Press and Bloomington, IN: Indiana University Press, 1998), 21–22.
89. Research participant Jenny, talking about text messages she receives, quoted in Christine Mellor, Deborah Payne and Judith McAra-Couper, 'Midwives' Perspectives of Maternal Mental Health Assessment and Screening for Risk during Pregnancy', *New Zealand College of Midwives Journal* 55 (1 December 2019): 27–34, 31.
90. A. S. Khashan, C. Everard, L. M. E. McCowan, G. Dekker, R. Moss-Morris, P. N. Baker, L. Poston, J. J. Walker, L. C. Kenny; the SCOPE Consortium, 'Second-Trimester Maternal Distress Increases the Risk of Small for Gestational Age', *Psychological Medicine* 44 (2014): 2799–2810; Sarah Rose, Gianella Pana and Shahirose Premji, 'Prenatal Maternal Anxiety as a Risk Factor for Preterm Birth and the Effects of Heterogeneity on This Relationship', *Biomed Research International* (2016); Aleksandra Staneva, Fiona Bogossian, Margo Pritchard and Anja Wittkowski, 'The Effects of Maternal Depression, Anxiety, and Perceived Stress during Pregnancy on Preterm Birth: A Systematic Review', *Women and Birth* 28, no. 3 (1 September 2015): 179–193.
91. Andrew Symon, Brian Williams, Qadir A. Adelasoye and Helen Cheyne, 'Nocebo and the Potential Harm of "High Risk" Labelling: A Scoping Review', *Journal of Advanced Nursing* 71, no.7 (July 2015): 1518–1529.
92. Carla Houkamau, David Tipene-Leach and Kathrine Clarke, 'The High Price of Being Labelled "High Risk": Social Context as a Health Determinant for Sudden Unexpected Infant Death in Māori Communities', *New Zealand College of Midwives Journal*, no. 52 (1 December 2016): 56–62.
93. Ibid., 58.

94. Ibid., 59.
95. See, for example, Ngā Maia Māori Midwives ō Aotearoa: 'Ngā Maia is committed to Māori birthing practices that promote the health and wellbeing of whānau.' *Ngā Maia Trust*, 'About Us', https://ngamaiatrust.org/home (last accessed May 2024); See also, Liza K. Edmonds, Fiona Cram, Matthew Bennett, Charlie Lambert, Anna Adcock, Kendall Stevenson, Stacie Geller, Evelyn Jane MacDonald, Tina Bennett, Francesca Storey, Melanie Gibson-Helm, Sidney Ropitini, Brittany Taylor, Victoria Bell, Caitlin Hoskin and Beverly Lawton, 'Hapū Ora (Pregnancy Wellness): Māori Research Responses From Conception, Through Pregnancy and "the First 1000 Days"–A Call to Action For Us All', *Journal of the Royal Society of New Zealand* 52, no. 4 (2022): 318–334.
96. On risk as a 'scare tactic', see Mariamni Plested and Mavis Kirkham, 'Risk and Fear in the Lived Experience of Birth Without a Midwife', *Midwifery* 38 (2016): 29–34, 29.
97. Ibid., 31.
98. Mari Greenfield, Sophie Payne-Gifford and Gemma McKenzie, 'Between a Rock and a Hard Place: Considering 'Freebirth' During Covid-19', *Frontiers in Global Women's Health*, 2 (18 February 2021): 10.
99. A. J. McMichael, 'Prisoners of the Proximate: Loosening the Constraints on Epidemiology in an Age of Change', *American Journal of Epidemiology* 149, no. 10 (15 May 1999): 887–897.
100. Weir, *Pregnancy, Risk and Biopolitics*, 58.
101. Ibid.
102. Howard Waitzkin, 'A Marxist View of Medical Care', *Annals of Internal Medicine* 89, no. 2 (1 August 1978): 264–278, 264.
103. H. I. Brumberg, H. L. and S. I. Shah, 'Born Early and Born Poor: An Eco-Bio-Developmental Model for Poverty and Preterm Birth', *Journal of Neonatal-Perinatal Medicine* 8, no. 3 (1 January 2015): 179–87; Emily A. DeFranco, Min Lian, Louis A. Muglia and Mario Schootman, 'Area-Level Poverty and Preterm Birth Risk: A Population-Based Multilevel Analysis', *BMC Public Health* 8 (2008): 316; Carol Kingdon, Devender Roberts, Mark A. Turner, Claire Storey, Nicola Crossland, Kenneth William Finlayson and Soo Downe, 'Inequalities and Stillbirth in the UK: A Meta-Narrative Review', *BMJ Open* 9, no. 9 (1 September 2019): e029672.
104. See, for example, Philip Blumenshine, Susan Egerter, Colleen J. Barclay, Catherine Cubbin and Paula A. Braveman, 'Socioeconomic Disparities in Adverse Birth Outcomes: A Systematic Review', *American Journal of Preventive Medicine* 39, no. 3 (1 September 2010): 263–272; A. Lindquist, N. Noor, E. Sullivan and M. Knight, 'The Impact of Socioeconomic Position on Severe Maternal Morbidity Outcomes among Women in Australia: A National Case-Control Study', *BJOG: An International Journal of Obstetrics & Gynaecology* 122, no. 12 (November 2015): 1601–1609.
105. McMichael, 'Prisoners of the Proximate'.

CHAPTER 5 THE GOLD STANDARD OF EVIDENCE

1. Cochrane, '1931–1971: A Critical Review with Particular Reference to the Medical Profession'.

2. Wendland, 'The Vanishing Mother', 228.
3. Andrea Ford, 'Advocating for Evidence in Birth: Proving Cause, Effecting Outcomes, and the Case for "Curers"', *Medicine Anthropology Theory* 6, no. 2 (2019): 25–48, 29.
4. Sara Wickham, 'Seeing Women in the Numbers', *MIDIRS Midwifery Digest* 13, no. 4 (2003): 439–444, 439.
5. David S. Jones and Scott H. Podolsky, 'The History and Fate of the Gold Standard', *The Lancet* 385, no. 9977 (18 April 2015): 1502–1503.
6. Ibid., 1502.
7. Mary E. Hannah, Walter J. Hannah, Sheila A. Hewson, Ellen D. Hodnett, Saroj Saigal and Andrew R. Willan, 'Planned Caesarean Section versus Planned Vaginal Birth for Breech Presentation at Term: A Randomised Multicentre Trial', *The Lancet* 356, no. 9239 (21 October 2000): 1375–1383.
8. Navarro, 'Professional Dominance or Proletarianization? Neither'.
9. Viviane Quirke, 'The Material Culture of British Pharmaceutical Laboratories in the Golden Age of Drug Discovery', *International Journal for the History of Engineering & Technology* 79 (2009): 280–299.
10. Ibid., 296.
11. 'Thalidomide', *Science Museum* (London), 11 December 2019, https://tinyurl.com/vzs3bf8p (last accessed May 2024).
12. Suzanne Junod, 'FDA and Clinical Drug Trials: A Short History', *FDLI Update* 2008, no. 2 (March/April 2008): 55–57; Stefan Timmermans and Marc Berg, *The Gold Standard: The Challenge of Evidence-Based Medicine and Standardization in Health Care* (Philadelphia, PA: Temple University Press, 2003), 89–90.
13. John Concato and Ralph I. Horwitz, 'Randomized Trials and Evidence in Medicine: A Commentary on Deaton and Cartwright', *Social Science & Medicine* 210 (August 2018): 32–36, 32.
14. Ernest Mandel, *Power and Money: A Marxist Theory of Bureaucracy* (London and New York: Verso, 1992), 154.
15. Andreas Lundh, Joel Lexchin, Barbara Mintzes, Jeppe B. Schroll and Lisa Bero, 'Industry Sponsorship and Research Outcome', *Cochrane Database of Systematic Reviews* 2017, Issue 2, Art. No.: MR000033 (last accessed May 2024).
16. Cochrane, '1931–1971: A Critical Review with Particular Reference to the Medical Profession', 10.
17. Ibid., 11.
18. Wagner, *Pursuing the Birth Machine*, 21.
19. Ibid., 20–21.
20. Ana Fernandez, Joachim Sturmberg, Sue Lukersmith, Rosamond Madden, Ghazal Torkfar, Ruth Colagiuri and Luis Salvador-Carulla, 'Evidence-Based Medicine: Is It a Bridge Too Far?' *Health Research Policy and Systems* 13, no. 1 (2015): 66, 3 of 9.
21. Concato and Horwitz, 'Randomized Trials and Evidence in Medicine', 32.
22. 'About the Cochrane Library', *Cochrane Library*, www.cochranelibrary.com/about/about-cochrane-library (last accessed May 2024).
23. 'Cochrane Central Register of Controlled Trials (CENTRAL)', *Cochrane Library*, www.cochranelibrary.com/central/about-central (last accessed May 2024).

24. 'About Cochrane Reviews', *Cochrane Library*, www.cochranelibrary.com/about/about-cochrane-reviews#:~:text=What%20is%20a%20systematic%20review,answer%20a%20specific%20research%20question (last accessed May 2024).
25. J. T. Hart, 'Cochrane Lecture 1997. What Evidence Do We Need for Evidence Based Medicine?' *Journal of Epidemiology & Community Health* 51, no. 6 (1997): 623–629, 623–624.
26. Cochrane, *Effectiveness and Efficiency*, 4.
27. Ibid., 12.
28. Hart, 'Cochrane Lecture 1997. What Evidence Do We Need for Evidence Based Medicine?', 623–624.
29. Ibid., 624.
30. Barbara Katz Rothman, 'Caught in the Current', in *Consuming Motherhood*, eds Janelle S. Taylor, Linda L. Layne and Danielle F. Wozniak (New Brunswick, NJ and London: Rutgers University Press, 2004), 279–288, 283.
31. Benjamin Djulbegovic and Gordon H. Guyatt, 'Progress in Evidence-Based Medicine: A Quarter Century On', *The Lancet* 390, no. 10092 (2017): 415–423, 417.
32. For information on cohort studies, see Aaron Kandola, 'Cohort Studies: What are They, Examples and Types', *Medical New Today*, updated 25 April 2023, www.medicalnewstoday.com/articles/281703. For information on case-control studies, see Susan Lewallen and Paul Courtright, 'Epidemiology in Practice: Case-Control Studies', *Community Eye Health* 11, 28 (1998): 57–58.
33. Sydney Pettygrove, 'Randomization', in *Encyclopedia of Epidemiology*, ed. Sarah Boslaugh (Los Angeles, CA: SAGE Publications, Inc., 2007, online 2012).
34. Paul J. Karanicolas, Forough Farrokhyar and Mohit Bhandari, 'Blinding: Who, What, When, Why, How?', *Canadian Journal of Surgery* 53, no. 5 (October 2010): 345–348.
35. Josiane Bonnefoy, Antony Morgan, Michael P. Kelly, Jennifer Butt and Vivian Bergman, *Constructing the Evidence Base on the Social Determinants of Health: A Guide*, Facultaci de Medicine (Universidad del Desarrollo) and National Institute for Health and Clinical Excellence, November 2007, 28.
36. Alfred Sohn-Rethel, *Intellectual and Manual Labour: A Critique of Epistemology* (London and Basingstoke: The Macmillan Press Ltd., 1978), 131–132.
37. Ibid., 132.
38. Ibid., 132.
39. Ibid., 131–132.
40. Nancy Cartwright, 'What Are Randomised Controlled Trials Good For?' *Philosophical Studies* 147, no. 1 (1 October 2009): 59–70.
41. Ian J. Saldanha, Andrea C. Skelly, Kelly Vander Ley, Zhen Wang, Elise Berliner, Eric B. Bass, Beth Devine, Noah Hammarlund, Gaelen P. Adam, Denise Duan-Porter, Lionel L. Bañez, Anjali Jain, Susan L. Norris, Timothy J. Wilt, Brian Leas, Shazia M. Siddique, Celia V. Fiordalisi, Cecilia Patino-Sutton and Meera Viswanathan, *Inclusion of Nonrandomized Studies of Interventions in Systematic Reviews of Intervention Effectiveness: An Update* (Rockville, MD: Agency for Healthcare Research and Quality, September 2022), 5, https://effectivehealthcare.ahrq.gov/sites/default/files/product/pdf/methods-guide-inclusion-nonrandomized-studies.pdf (last accessed May 2024).

42. Hannah et al., 'Planned Caesarean Section versus Planned Vaginal Birth for Breech Presentation at Term.'
43. Ibid.
44. Catherine Y. Spong, 'Defining "Term" Pregnancy: Recommendations From the Defining "Term" Pregnancy Workgroup', *JAMA* 309, no. 23 (19 June 2013): 2445–2446.
45. Jacana Bresson, Keelie Christie and Shawn Walker, 'Not Too Fast, Not Too Slow: A Review of Historical Trends in Vaginal Breech Time Management', *European Journal of Obstetrics & Gynecology and Reproductive Biology* 287 (2023): 216–220.
46. Deidre Spelliscy Gifford, Sally C. Morton, Mary Fiske and Katherine Kahn, 'A Meta-Analysis of Infant Outcomes After Breech Delivery', *Obstetrics & Gynecology* 85, no. 6 (1 June 1995): 1047–1054; Josefin Roman, Oddvar Bakos and Sven Cnattingius, 'Pregnancy Outcomes by Mode of Delivery Among Term Breech Births: Swedish Experience 1987–1993', *Obstetrics & Gynecology* 92, no. 6 (1998): 945–950.
47. Hannah et al., 'Planned Caesarean Section versus Planned Vaginal Birth for Breech Presentation at Term', 1381.
48. For more precise description of the criteria for participation in the trial, see ibid., 1375–1376.
49. The study was stopped earlier than originally had been anticipated. In the words of the primary investigators, 'After reviewing the results of the second interim analysis, the data monitoring committee recommended that recruitment be stopped, since the difference in the rate of the primary outcome between groups was significant at p<0·002. Recruitment was stopped the following day on April 21, 2000.' Ibid., 1378.
50. Ibid., 1375.
51. Ibid., 1375.
52. See, for example, Gerald W. Lawson, 'The Term Breech Trial Ten Years on: Primum Non Nocere?' *Birth* 39, no. 1 (2012): 3–9; Marek Glezerman, 'Five Years to the Term Breech Trial: The Rise and Fall of a Randomized Controlled Trial', *American Journal of Obstetrics and Gynecology* 194, no. 1 (1 January 2006): 20–25.
53. Kotaska Andrew, 'Inappropriate Use of Randomised Trials to Evaluate Complex Phenomena: Case Study of Vaginal Breech Delivery', *British Medical Journal* 329, no. 7473 (2004): 1039–1042, 1040.
54. Ibid., 1041.
55. Ibid., 1041.
56. Ibid., 1040.
57. See, for example, David Somerset, 'Term Breech Trial Does Not Provide Unequivocal Evidence (Letter)', *British Medical Journal* 324, no. 7328 (2002): 49.
58. Enkin et al., 'Beyond Evidence: The Complexity of Maternity Care', 267.
59. Nancy Cartwright, 'What Are Randomised Controlled Trials Good For?' *Philosophical Studies* 147, no.1 (1 October 2009): 59–70, 65.
60. Angus Deaton and Nandy Cartwright, 'Understanding and Misunderstanding Randomized Controlled Trials', *Social Science & Medicine* 210 (2018): 2–21, 17.

61. For discussion of the subgroup analysis carried out in the Term Breech Trial, see Kotaska, 'Inappropriate Use of Randomised Trials to Evaluate Complex Phenomena', 1040.
62. Hannah et al., 'Planned Caesarean Section versus Planned Vaginal Birth for Breech Presentation at Term', 1375.
63. Ibid., 1382.
64. Kotaska, 'Inappropriate Use of Randomised Trials to Evaluate Complex Phenomena', 1040.
65. Ibid., 1041.
66. Ibid.
67. Glezerman, 'Five Years to the Term Breech Trial', 20.
68. Betty-Anne Daviss, Kenneth C. Johnson and André B. Lalonde, 'Evolving Evidence since the Term Breech Trial: Canadian Response, European Dissent, and Potential Solutions', *Journal of Obstetrics and Gynaecology Canada* 32, no. 3 (2010): 217–224.
69. Christine C. Th. Rietberg, Patty M. Elferink-Stinkens and Gerard H. A. Visser, 'The Effect of the Term Breech Trial on Medical Intervention Behaviour and Neonatal Outcome in The Netherlands: An Analysis of 35,453 Term Breech Infants', *BJOG* 112, no. 2 (2005): 205–209.
70. Sara Morris, Sadie Geraghty and Deborah Sundin, 'Moxibustion: An Alternative Option for Breech Presentation', *British Journal of Midwifery* 26, no. 7 (2018): 440–445.
71. Shawn Walker, Emma Spillane, Kate Stringer, Amy Meadowcroft, Tisha Dasgupta, Siân M. Davies, Jane Sandall, Andrew Shennan and the OptiBreech Collaborative, 'The Feasibility of Team Care for Women Seeking to Plan a Vaginal Breech Birth (OptiBreech 1): An Observational Implementation Feasibility Study in Preparation for a Pilot Trial', *Pilot and Feasibility Studies* 9, no. 1 (2023): 80.
72. Amos Grunebaum, 'Vaginal Breech Deliveries in the United States: 1999–2013 [14H]', *Obstetrics & Gynecology* 127 (May 2016): 69S–70S.
73. Mark P. Hehir, 'Trends in Vaginal Breech Delivery', *Journal of Epidemiology and Community Health* 69 (2015): 1237–1239; Mark P. Hehir, Hugh D. O'Connor, Etaoin M. Kent, Chris Fitzpatrick, Peter C. Boylan, Samuel Coulter-Smith, Michael P. Geary and Fergal D. Malone, 'Changes in Vaginal Breech Delivery Rates in a Single Large Metropolitan Area', *American Journal of Obstetrics and Gynecology* 206, no. 6 (2012): 498.e1–498.e4.
74. Roberto Palencia, Amiram Gafni, Mary E. Hannah, Susan Ross, Andrew R. Willan, Sheila Hewson, Darren McKay, Walter Hannah, Hilary Whyte, Kofi Amankwah, Mary Cheng, Patricia Guselle, Michael Helewa, Ellen D. Hodnett, Eileen K. Hutton, Rose Kung, Saroj Saigal, and for the Term Breech Trial Collaborative Group, 'The Costs of Planned Cesarean versus Planned Vaginal Birth in the Term Breech Trial', *Canadian Medical Association Journal* 174, no. 8 (11 April 2006): 1109–1113.
75. See, for example, Steven M. Rock, 'Malpractice Premiums and Primary Caesarean Section Rates in New York and Illinois', *Public Health Reports* 103, no. 5 (1988): 459–463, 460; Philip Zwecker, Laurent Azoulay and Haim A. Abenhaim, 'Effect of Fear of Litigation on Obstetric Care: A Nationwide Analysis on Obstetric Practice', *American Journal of Perinatology* 28, no. 4

(2011): 277–284, 278; See also Glezerman, 'Five Years to the Term Breech Trial', 24.

76. Glezerman, 'Five Years to the Term Breech Trial', 24.
77. Marc J. N. C. Keirse, 'Evidence-Based Childbirth Only For Breech Babies?' *Birth* 29, no. 1 (2002): 55–59, 56.
78. M. J. Turner, 'The Term Breech Trial: Are the Clinical Guidelines Justified by the Evidence?' *Journal of Obstetrics and Gynaecology* 26, no. 6 (2006): 491–494, 492.
79. Andrew Kotaska, 'Commentary: Routine Cesarean Section for Breech: The Unmeasured Cost', *Birth* 38, no. 2 (June 2011): 162–164, 162.
80. Andrew Ure, *The Philosophy of Manufactures*, quoted in Marx, *Capital, Volume 1*, 559–560.
81. Harry Braverman, *Labor and Monopoly Capital: The Degradation of Work in the Twentieth Century* (New York: Monthly Review Press, 25th Anniversary Edition, Digital, 1998), 356.
82. Hilary Whyte, Mary E. Hannah, Saroj Saigal, Walter J. Hannah, Sheila Hewson, Kofi Amankwah, Mary Cheng, Amiram Gafni, Patricia Guselle, Michael Helewa, Ellen D. Hodnett, Eileen Hutton, Rose Kung, Darren McKay, Susan Ross and Andrew Willan for the 2-year Infant Follow-up Term Breech Trial Collaborative Group, 'Outcomes of Children at 2 Years after Planned Cesarean Birth versus Planned Vaginal Birth for Breech Presentation at Term: The International Randomized Term Breech Trial', *American Journal of Obstetrics and Gynecology* 191, no. 3 (2004): 864–871.
83. Andrew Kotaska and Savas Menticoglou, 'No. 384-Management of Breech Presentation at Term', *Journal of Obstetrics and Gynaecology Canada* 41, no. 8 (1 August 2019): 1193–1205, 1197.
84. François Goffinet, Marion Carayol, Jean-Michel Foidart, Sophie Alexander, Serge Uzan, Damien Subtil and Gérard Bréart, 'Is Planned Vaginal Delivery for Breech Presentation at Term Still an Option? Results of an Observational Prospective Survey in France and Belgium', *American Journal of Obstetrics and Gynecology* 194, no. 4 (1 April 2006): 1002–1011.
85. Ibid., 1003.
86. Betty-Anne Daviss, Kenneth C. Johnson, and André B. Lalonde, 'Evolving Evidence since the Term Breech Trial: Canadian Response, European Dissent, and Potential Solutions', *Journal of Obstetrics and Gynaecology Canada* 32, no. 3 (2010): 217–224, 217.
87. Mark P. Hehir, 'Trends in Vaginal Breech Delivery', *Journal of Epidemiology and Community Health* 69 (2015): 1237–1239, 1237–1238.
88. Andrew Kotaska, 'Commentary: Routine Cesarean Section for Breech: The Unmeasured Cost', *Birth* 38, no. 2 (June 2011): 162–164; Joke M. Schutte, Eric A. P. Steegers, Job G. Santema, Nico W. E. Schuitemaker and Jos Van Roosmalen, 'Maternal Deaths After Elective Cesarean Section for Breech Presentation in the Netherlands', *Acta Obstetricia et Gynecologica Scandinavica* 86, no. 2 (2007): 240–243; Sabrina Das, 'Resurrecting a Lost Obstetric Skill to Reduce Global Maternal Death', *BMJ Global Health Blogs*, 10 February 2023, https://blogs.bmj.com/bmjgh/2023/02/10/resurrecting-a-lost-obstetric-skill-to-reduce-global-maternal-death/ (last accessed May 2024).

89. Karolina Petrovska, Nicole P. Watts, Christine Catling, Andrew Bisits and Caroline S. E. Homer. '"Stress, Anger, Fear and Injustice": An International Qualitative Survey of Women's Experiences Planning a Vaginal Breech Birth', *Midwifery* 44 (2017): 41–47.
90. See, for example, 'Breech Without Borders', *Breech Without Borders*, www.breechwithoutborders.org/ (last accessed May 2024); Jane Evans, 'Breech Birth', in *Normalizing Challenging or Complex Childbirth*, eds Karen Jackson and Helen Wightman (Open University Press & McGraw Hill Education, Kindle Education, 2017).
91. James Erskine, 'Term Breech Trial: Letter', *The Lancet* 357, no. 9251 (20 January 2001): 228.
92. Sabrina Das, 'Resurrecting a Lost Obstetric Skill to Reduce Global Maternal Death'.
93. For an interesting discussion of some of the limitations of RCTs, see Kenneth C. Johnson, 'Randomized Controlled Trials as Authoritative Knowledge: Keeping an Ally from Becoming a Threat to North American Midwifery Practice', in *Childbirth and Authoritative Knowledge: Cross-Cultural Perspectives*, eds Robbie E. Davis-Floyd and Carolyn F. Sargent (California and London: University of California Press, 1997 [E-book]).
94. Angus Deaton and Nancy Cartwright, 'Reflections on Randomized Control Trials', *Social Science & Medicine* 210 (August 2018): 86–90, 86.
95. William A. Grobman, Madeline M. Rice, Uma M. Reddy, Alan T. N. Tita, Robert M. Silver, Gail Mallett, Kim Hill, Elizabeth A. Thom, Yasser Y. El-Sayed, Annette Perez-Delboy, Dwight J. Rouse, George R. Saade, Kim A. Boggess, Suneet P. Chauhan, Jay D. Iams, Edward K. Chien, Brian M. Casey, Ronald S. Gibbs, Sindhu K. Srinivas, Geeta K. Swamy, Hyagriv N. Simhan and George A. Macones, 'Labor Induction versus Expectant Management in Low-Risk Nulliparous Women', *New England Journal of Medicine* 379, no. 6 (9 August 2018): 513–523; Miranda Davies-Tuck, Euan M. Wallace and Caroline S. E. Homer, 'Why ARRIVE Should Not Thrive in Australia', *Women and Birth* 31, no. 5 (1 October 2018): 339–340; Fabio Facchinetti, Daniela Menichini and Enrica Perrone, 'The ARRIVE Trial Will Not "Arrive" to Europe', *Journal of Maternal-Fetal & Neonatal Medicine* 35, no. 22 (2020): 4229–4232; 'Research Debates: The Arrive Trial – Should It Influence Practice in New Zealand?' *New Zealand College of Midwives*, www.midwife.org.nz/midwives/research/research-debates/ (last accessed May 2024); Beatrice M. G. Tassis, Marta Ruggiero, Alice Ronchi, Ilaria G. Ramezzana, Giulia Bischetti, Enrico Iurlaro, Francesco D'Ambrosi, Fabrizio Ciralli, Fabio Mosca and Enrico M. Ferrazzi, 'An Hypothetical External Validation of the ARRIVE Trial in a European Academic Hospital', *Journal of Maternal-Fetal & Neonatal Medicine* 35, no. 2 (18 November 2020): 4291–4298.
96. Vivienne Souter, Elizabeth Nethery, Barbara Levy, Kate Mclean and Kristin Sitcov, 'Elective Induction of Labor in Nulliparas: Has the ARRIVE Trial Changed Obstetric Practices and Outcomes?' *American Journal of Obstetrics & Gynecology* 226, no. 1 (2022): S83–S84.
97. See, for example, Helen Barratt, Marion Campbell, Laurence Moore, Merrick Zwarenstein and Peter Bower, 'Randomised Controlled Trials of Complex Interventions and Large-Scale Transformation of Services', in Rosalind Raine,

Ray Fitzpatrick, Helen Barratt, Gywn Bevan, Nick Black and Ruth Boaden et al., 'Challenges, Solutions and Future Directions in the Evaluation of Service Innovations in Health Care and Public Health', *Health Services and Delivery Research* 4, no. 16 (2016): 19–36; Ann Oakley, Vicki Strange, Chris Bonell, Elizabeth Allen and Judith Stephenson, 'Process Evaluation in Randomised Controlled Trials of Complex Interventions', *BMJ* 332, no. 7538 (2006): 413–416.

98. Djulbegovic and Guyatt, 'Progress in Evidence-Based Medicine'.
99. Ibid.
100. Reed Siemieniuk and Gordon Guyatt, 'What is GRADE?' *British Medical Journal Best Practice*, https://bestpractice.bmj.com/info/toolkit/learn-ebm/what-is-grade/ (last accessed May 2024).
101. David L. Sackett, William M. C. Rosenberg, J. A. Muir Gray, R. Brian Haynes, and W. Scott Richardson, 'Evidence Based Medicine: What It Is and What It Isn't', *BMJ* 312, no. 7023 (13 January 1996): 71–72, 71.
102. Sheryl Burt Ruzek, 'Defining Reducible Risk: Social Dimensions of Assessing Birth Technologies', *Human Nature* 4, no. 4 (1993): 383–408, 401.
103. On the first point, see Billie F. Bradford, Alyce N. Wilson, Anayda Portela, Fran McConville, Cristina Fernandez Turienzo and Caroline S. E. Homer, 'Midwifery Continuity of Care: A Scoping Review of Where, How, By Whom and For Whom?' *PLOS Global Public Health* 2, no. 10 (2022), e0000935. They note that 'With the exception of New Zealand, no countries have managed to scale-up continuity of midwifery care at a national level.' Regarding clinical guidelines, see, for example, K. Prusova, L. Churcher, A. Tyler and A. U. Lokugamage, 'Royal College of Obstetricians and Gynaecologists Guidelines: How Evidence-based are They?' *Journal of Obstetrics and Gynaecology* 34, no. 8 (2014): 706–711.
104. Robbie Davis-Floyd, *Birth as an American Rite of Passage* (London and New York: Routledge, 2022, 3rd edition), xxii & 74.
105. Fredric Jameson, *Representing Capital: A Reading of Volume 1* (Verso, 2014, ebook edition), Introduction, paragraph 12.

CHAPTER 6 FREEDOM OF CHOICE?

1. Abby Lippman, 'Choice as a Risk to Women's Health', *Health, Risk & Society* 1, no. 3 (1 November 1999): 281–291, 281.
2. Karl Marx, 'The Eighteenth Brumaire of Louis Bonaparte', in *Marx: Later Political Writings*, ed. and trans. Terrell Carver (Cambridge University Press, 1996), 31–127, 32. These words of Marx were also drawn upon by political scientist, Rosalind Pollack Petchesky, in her discussion of reproductive freedom especially in relation to birth control, abortion and childcare. Rosalind Pollack Petchesky, 'Reproductive Freedom: Beyond "A Woman's Right to Choose"', *Signs: Journal of Women in Culture and Society* 5, no. 4 (July 1980): 661–685, 675.
3. See, for example, Karl Marx, *Economic and Philosophic Manuscripts of 1844*, trans. Martin Milligan (Start Publishing LLC, Kindle Edition, 2012): 73–76.
4. Ibid., 75.
5. Ibid.

6. See, for example, ibid., 74–76.
7. Ibid., 71.
8. Marx and Engels, *The German Ideology*, 41.
9. Marx, *Economic and Philosophic Manuscripts of 1844*, 73.
10. Ibid., 100–101.
11. '... the art of midwifery is, in the hands of men, like certain plants, which, by dint of a forcing culture, exhibit more florish, or a broader expansion; but besides ever retaining a certain exotic appearance, they never come up to the virtue of those spontaneously growing in the full vigor of a soil of nature's own choice for them.' Elizabeth Nihell, *A Treatise on the Art of Midwifery*, 105.
12. Hannah Rion, *The Truth About Twilight Sleep* (New York: McBride, Nast & Company, 1915), 56.
13. Ibid., 56.
14. Fraser, 'Contradictions of Capital and Care', 104.
15. Lippman, 'Choice as a Risk to Women's Health', 282.
16. Beverley Beech, '50 Years' Campaigning' (introductory speech at the 50th Anniversary Luncheon, 16 October 2010), *AIMS Journal* 22, no. 4 (2010), www.aims.org.uk/journal/item/50-years-campaigning (last accessed May 2024).
17. House of Commons Health Committee, *Second Report on the Maternity Services* (London: HMSO, 1992); Department of Health, *Changing Childbirth: Report of the Expert Maternity Group (Chair Julia Cumberlege)* (London: HMSO, 1993); Department of Health/Partnerships for Children, Families and Maternity, *Maternity Matters: Choice, Access and Continuity of Care in a Safe Service* (London: Department of Health, April 2007).
18. Alicia O'Cathain, 'Can Leaflets Deliver Informed Choice?' in *Informed Choice in Maternity Care*, ed. Mavis Kirkham (London and New York: Palgrave Macmillan, 2004), 71–85.
19. Committee of Inquiry into Allegations Concerning the Treatment of Cervical Cancer at National Women's Hospital and into Other Related Matters, *The Report of the Cervical Cancer Inquiry* (Auckland, New Zealand, July 1988).
20. 'The Cartwright Inquiry', *Women's Health Action*, www.womens-health.org.nz/the-cartwright-inquiry/ (last accessed May 2024).
21. Rothman, 'Caught in the Current', 283.
22. Christa Craven, 'A "Consumer's Right" to Choose a Midwife: Shifting Meanings for Reproductive Rights under Neoliberalism', *American Anthropologist* 109, no. 4 (2007): 701–712.
23. Karl Marx, *A Contribution to the Critique of Political Economy*, trans. S. W. Ryazanskaya (London: Lawrence & Wishart, 1971), 206.
24. Sheila Kitzinger, *Freedom and Choice in Childbirth* (London: Penguin Books, 1988), 273.
25. Tricia Anderson and Jilly Rosser, 'Informed Choice: Was It the Wrong Choice?' *The Practising Midwife* 1, no. 10 (1998): 4–5.
26. Ibid., 4.
27. Tricia Anderson, 'No More Consumers, Please', *The Practising Midwife* 9, no. 7 (2006): 51.
28. Adam Smith, *The Wealth of Nations: Books IV–V*, ed. Andrew Skinner (Middlesex, England: Penguin Books, 1999, Digital Edition) [Book IV, Part III. Of the Expense of Public Works and Public Institutions].

29. Anderson, 'No More Consumers, Please', 51.
30. Ruth Sanders and Kenda Crozier, 'How Do Informal Information Sources Influence Women's Decision-Making for Birth? A Meta-Synthesis of Qualitative Studies', *BMC Pregnancy and Childbirth* 18 (10 January 2018): 21.
31. Anderson, 'No More Consumers, Please', 51.
32. G. A. Skowronski, 'Pain Relief in Childbirth: Changing Historical and Feminist Perspectives'', *Anaesthesia and Intensive Care* 43 (Historical Supplement): 25–28, 25.
33. Ronald Melzack, 'The Myth of Painless Childbirth (The John J. Bonica Lecture)', *Pain* 19, no. 4 (August 1984).
34. Leap, 'Being with Women in Pain – Do Midwives Need to Rethink Their Role?' *British Journal of Midwifery* 5, no. 5 (1997): 263.
35. Ibid.
36. For discussion of Melzack and Wall's Gate Control Theory, see Linda Wylie, *Essential Anatomy and Physiology in Maternity Care* (Churchill Livingstone, 2002), 27.
37. Sarah J. Buckley, 'Executive Summary of Hormonal Physiology of Childbearing: Evidence and Implications for Women, Babies, and Maternity Care', *Journal of Perinatal Education* 24, no. 3 (2015): 145–153, 149 and 150.
38. Van der Gucht, Natalie and Kiara Lewis, 'Women's Experiences of Coping with Pain during Childbirth: A Critical Review of Qualitative Research', *Midwifery* 31, no. 3 (2015): 349–358, 352.
39. Research participant, Susan, quoted in Sigridur Halldorsdottir and Sigfridur Inga Karlsdottir, 'Journeying through Labour and Delivery: Perceptions of Women Who Have Given Birth', *Midwifery* 12, no. 2 (1996): 48–61, 53.
40. Research participant, Sharon, quoted in Nicky Leap, Jane Sandall, Sara Buckland and Ulli Huber, 'Journey to Confidence: Women's Experiences of Pain in Labour and Relational Continuity of Care', *Journal of Midwifery & Women's Health* 55, no. 3 (2010): 234–242, 239.
41. Bogod, 'Epidural Denial. Thoughts from the Frontline'.
42. Ibid.
43. Penny Curtis, Linda Ball and Mavis Kirkham, 'Why Do Midwives Leave? (Not) Being the Kind of Midwife You Want to Be'; Royal College of Midwives, *Why Midwives Leave – Revisited. British Journal of Midwifery* 14, no. 1 (January 2006): 27–31.
44. See, for example, Alyssa Knox, Geneviève Rouleau, Sonia Semenic, Malisa Khongkham, and Luisa Ciofani, 'Barriers and Facilitators to Birth without Epidural in a Tertiary Obstetric Referral Center: Perspectives of Health Care Professionals and Patients', *Birth* 45, no. 3 (2018): 295–302.
45. Theresa Morris and Mia Schulman, 'Race Inequality in Epidural Use and Regional Anesthesia Failure in Labor and Birth: An Examination of Women's Experience', *Sexual & Reproductive Healthcare* 5, no. 4 (2014): 188–194, 189.
46. Alexander J. Butwick, Jason Bentley, Cynthia A. Wong, Jonathan M. Snowden, Eric Sun and Nan Guo, 'United States State-Level Variation in the Use of Neuraxial Analgesia During Labor for Pregnant Women', *JAMA Network Open* 1, no. 8 (7 December 2018): e186567–e186567.
47. Mavis Kirkham and Helen Stapleton, 'Chapter 16: The Culture of Maternity Care', in *Informed Choice in Maternity Care: An Evaluation of Evidence Based*

Leaflets, eds Mavis Kirkham and Helen Stapleton (NHS Centre for Reviews and Dissemination, The University of York, Report 20, 2001): 137–150, 140.

48. Ibid.
49. Ibid.
50. Ibid.
51. Research participants quoted in Dana A. Schneider, 'Birthing Failures: Childbirth as a Female Fault Line', *Journal of Perinatal Education* 27, no. 1 (2018): 20–31, 24.
52. Birthrights, *Maternal Request Caesarean* (UK: Birthrights, August 2018), https://birthrights.org.uk/wp-content/uploads/2018/08/Final-Birthrights-MRCS-Report-2108-1.pdf (last accessed May 2024).
53. Jane Weaver and Julia Magill-Cuerden, '"Too Posh to Push": The Rise and Rise of a Catchphrase', *Birth* 40, no. 4 (December 2013): 264–271.
54. Ibid., 266.
55. Katherine Beckett, 'Choosing Cesarean: Feminism and the Politics of Childbirth in the United States', *Feminist Theory* 6, no. 3 (2005): 251–75, 251.
56. Kristiane Tislevoll Eide, Nils-Halvdan Morken and Kristine Bærøe, 'Maternal Reasons for Requesting Planned Cesarean Section in Norway: A Qualitative Study', *BMC Pregnancy and Childbirth* 19, no. 102 (2019).
57. Charles O'Donovan and James O'Donovan, 'Why Do Women Request an Elective Cesarean Delivery for Non-Medical Reasons? A Systematic Review of the Qualitative Literature', *Birth* 45, no. 2 (2018): 109–119; Eide, Morken, and Bærøe, 'Maternal Reasons for Requesting Planned Cesarean Section in Norway'.
58. See, for example, Rachel Reed, Rachael Sharman and Christian Inglis, 'Women's Descriptions of Childbirth Trauma Relating to Care Provider Actions and Interactions', *BMC Pregnancy and Childbirth* 17, no. 21 (10 January 2017); Jenny Patterson, Caroline J. Hollins Martin and Thanos Karatzias, 'Disempowered Midwives and Traumatised Women: Exploring the Parallel Processes of Care Provider Interaction That Contribute to Women Developing Post Traumatic Stress Disorder (PTSD) Post Childbirth', *Midwifery* 76 (September 2019): 21–35; The All-Party Parliamentary Group on Birth Trauma, *Listen to Mums: Ending the Postcode Lottery in Perinatal Care, A report by The All-Party Parliamentary Group on Birth Trauma* (APPG, UK Parliament, May 2024).
59. Penny Curtis, Linda Ball and Mavis Kirkham, 'Bullying and Horizontal Violence: Cultural or Individual Phenomena?' *British Journal of Midwifery* 14, no. 4 (2006): 218–221.
60. Independent Maternity Review, *Ockenden Report – Final: Findings, Conclusions and Essential Actions from the Independent Review of Maternity Services at The Shrewsbury and Telford Hospital NHS Trust* (HC1219, Crown, 2022), https://assets.publishing.service.gov.uk/media/62433358d3bf7f32b317e8e5/Final-Ockenden-Report-print-ready.pdf (last accessed May 2024).
61. The All-Party Parliamentary Group on Birth Trauma, *Listen to Mums: Ending the Postcode Lottery on Perinatal Care.*
62. See, for example, Patterson et al., 'Disempowered Midwives and Traumatised Women'.

63. Tricia Anderson, 'The Misleading Myth of Choice: The Continuing Oppression of Women in Childbirth', in *Informed Choice in Maternity Care*, ed. Mavis Kirkham (London and New York: Palgrave Macmillan, 2004): 257–264, 264.
64. Rixa Freeze and Laura Tanner, 'Freebirth in the United States', in *Birthing Outside the System*, eds Hannah Dahlen, Bashi Kumar-Hazard and Virginia Schmied (Routledge, Taylor & Francis Group, 2020, E-book), 27–58, 33–34; Melanie Jackson, 'Giving Birth Outside the System in Australia: Freebirth and High-Risk Homebirth', in *Birthing Outside the System*, eds Hannah Dahlen, Bashi Kumar-Hazard and Virginia Schmied (Routledge, Taylor & Francis Group, 2020, E-book), 59–79, 61.
65. Gemma McKenzie, Glenn Robert and Elsa Montgomery, 'Exploring the Conceptualisation and Study of Freebirthing as a Historical and Social Phenomenon: A Meta-Narrative Review of Diverse Research Traditions', *Medical Humanities* 46, no. 4 (2020): 512–524, 518.
66. Tricia Anderson, 'The Misleading Myth of Choice: The Continuing Oppression of Women in Childbirth', 264.
67. Rebecca Schiller, 'The Women Hounded for Giving Birth Outside the System', *The Guardian*, 22 October 2016, www.theguardian.com/lifeandstyle/2016/oct/22/hounded-for-giving-birth-outside-the-system (last accessed May 2024).
68. See, for example, 'NHS Maternity Care and Charging', *Maternity Action*, https://maternityaction.org.uk/nhs-maternity-care-and-charging/ (last accessed July 2024).
69. Bridie Witton, 'More Women Unable to Afford Costly Pregnancy Scans', *Stuff*, 13 May 2024, www.stuff.co.nz/politics/350275705/more-women-unable-afford-costly-pregnancy-scans (last accessed July 2024).
70. Jordan Cahn, Ayesha Sundaram; Roopa Balachandar, Alexandra Berg, Aaron Birnbaum, Stephanie Hastings, Matthew Makansi, Emily Romano, Ariel Majidi, Danny McCormick and Adam Gaffney, 'The Association of Childbirth with Medical Debt, 2019–2020', *J Gen Intern Med.* 38, no. 10 (2023): 2340–2346.
71. Monica K. Miller, 'Refusal to Undergo a Cesarean Section: A Woman's Right or a Criminal Act?', *Health Matrix: The Journal of Law Medicine* 15, no. 2 (2005): 383–400; E. M. Dadlez and William L. Andrews, 'Not Separate, but Not Equal: How Fetal Rights Deprive Women of Civil Rights', *Public Affairs Quarterly* 26, no. 2 (2012): 103–122.
72. Lynn M. Paltrow and Jeanne Flavin, 'Arrests of and Forced Interventions on Pregnant Women in the United States, 1973–2005: Implications for Women's Legal Status and Public Health', *Journal of Health Politics, Policy and Law* 38, no. 2 (April 2013): 299–343.
73. Michele Goodwin, *Policing the Womb: Invisible Women and the Criminalization of Motherhood* (Cambridge: Cambridge University Press, Kindle Edition, 2020), 8.
74. Meghan Boone and Benjamin J. McMichael, 'State-Created Fetal Harm', *The Georgetown Law Journal* 109 (2021): 475–522, 475.
75. Goodwin, *Policing the Womb*, 191.
76. Tamar Sarai, 'Pregnancy, Parenthood, and Prison: The Right to Choose Where Autonomy is Illusive', *PRISM*, 19 July 2022, https://prismreports.org/2022/07/19/pregnancy-parenthood-prison-right-to-choose/ (last accessed May 2024).

77. Eugene Declercq, Ruby Barnard-Mayers, Laurie C. Zephyrin and Kay Johnson, 'The U.S. Maternal Health Divide: The Limited Maternal Health Services and Worse Outcomes of States Proposing New Abortion Restrictions', *The Commonwealth Fund*, 14 December 2022, www.commonwealthfund.org/publications/issue-briefs/2022/dec/us-maternal-health-divide-limited-services-worse-outcomes (last accessed May 2024).
78. Brittni Frederiksen, Usha Ranji, Ivette Gomez and Alina Salganicoff, *A National Survey of OBGYNs Experiences after Dobbs* (KFF, June 2023), https://files.kff.org/attachment/Report-A-National-Survey-of-OBGYNs-Experiences-After-Dobbs.pdf (last accessed May 2024).
79. 'Center Expands Work on Behalf of Patients Denied Abortion Care Despite Grave Pregnancy Complications', Center for Reproductive Rights, 12 September 2023, https://reproductiverights.org/exceptions-complaints-idaho-tennessee-oklahoma/ (last accessed May 2024); 'Texas Supreme Court Refuses to Clarify Abortion Ban Exceptions', Center for Reproductive Rights, 31 May 2024, https://reproductiverights.org/texas-supreme-court-refuses-to-clarify-abortion-ban-exceptions/ (last accessed June 2024).
80. Maggie Redshaw, Reem Malouf, Haiyan Gao and Ron Gray, 'Women with Disability: The Experience of Maternity Care During Pregnancy, Labour and Birth and the Postnatal Period', *BMC Pregnancy and Childbirth* 13, no. 1 (2013): 1–14; Birthrights, *Dignity in Childbirth: The Dignity Survey 2013: Women's and Midwives' Experiences of Dignity in UK Maternity Care* (Birthrights, 2013), https://birthrights.org.uk/wp-content/uploads/2013/10/Birthrights-Dignity-Survey-1.pdf; Jenny Hall, Vanora Hundley, Bethan Collins and Jillian Ireland, 'Dignity and Respect During Pregnancy and Childbirth: A Survey of the Experience of Disabled Women', *BMC Pregnancy and Childbirth* 18 (2018): 1–13.
81. Jasmina Cherguit, Jan Burns, Sharon Pettle and Fiona Tasker, 'Lesbian Co-mothers' Experiences of Maternity Healthcare Services', *Journal of Advanced Nursing* 69, no. 6 (2013): 1269–1278.
82. George Parker, Alex Ker, Sally Baddock, Elizabeth Kerekere, Jaimie Veale and Suzanne Miller, '"It's Total Erasure": Trans and Nonbinary Peoples' Experiences of Cisnormativity Within Perinatal Care Services in Aotearoa New Zealand', *Women's Reproductive Health*, 10, no. 4 (2023): 591–607; George Parker, Suzanne Miller, Sally Baddock, Jaimie Veale, Alex Ker and Elizabeth Kerekere, *Warming the Whare for Trans People and Whānau in Perinatal Care* (Otago Polytechnic Press, 2023); Alexis Hoffkling, Juno Obedin-Maliver and Jae Sevelius, 'From Erasure to Opportunity: A Qualitative Study of the Experiences of Transgender Men around Pregnancy and Recommendations for Providers', *BMC Pregnancy and Childbirth* 17, no. 322 (2017), 1–14.
83. George Parker et al., *Warming the Whare for Trans People and Whānau in Perinatal Care.*
84. Margaret Besse, Nik M. Lampe and Emily S. Mann, 'Experiences With Achieving Pregnancy and Giving Birth Among Transgender Men: A Narrative Literature Review', *Yale Journal of Biology and Medicine* 93, no. 4 (2020): 517–528.

85. Mari Greenfield, Sophie Payne-Gifford and Gemma McKenzie, 'Between a Rock and a Hard Place: Considering "Freebirth" During Covid-19', *Frontiers in Global Women's Health* 2, article 603744 (2021).
86. Mari Greenfield and Zoe Darwin, 'LGBTQ+ New and Expectant Parents' Experiences of Perinatal Services During the UK's First COVID-19 Lockdown', *Birth: Issues in Perinatal Care*, 51, no. 1 (2024): 134–144, 140.
87. '5/2/23 Member Communication: Cyclone Gabrielle', New Zealand College of Midwives, 15 February 2023, www.midwife.org.nz/news/15-2-23-member-communication-cyclone-gabrielle/ (last accessed May 2024); 'Babies Just Keep Being Born Even in a Natural Disaster', Hauora Taiwhenua Rural Health Network, 6 October 2023, https://htrhn.org.nz/news-media/babies-just-keep-being-born-even-in-a-natural-disaster/ (last accessed May 2024).
88. See, for example, Cara Baddington in 'Babies Just Keep Being Born Even in a Natural Disaster'.
89. See, for example, Jason W. Moore, ed., *Anthropocene or Capitalocene? Nature, History, and the Crisis of Capitalism* (Oakland, CA: PM Press, 2016).
90. See, for example, Carl Cassegård, *Toward a Critical Theory of Nature: Capital, Ecology, and Dialectics* (Bloomsbury Academic, 2021): 7.
91. 'G20 Countries Failing by Big Margins to Cut Greenhouse Gas Emission to Below "Catastrophic" Levels', *Oxfam International*, 7 September 2023, www.oxfam.org/en/press-releases/g20-countries-failing-big-margins-cut-greenhouse-gas-emissions-below-catastrophic (last accessed May 2024).
92. Alex Maitland, Max Lawson, Hilde Stroot, Alexandre Poidatz, Ashfaq Khalfan and Nafkote Dabi, *Carbon Billionaires: The Investment Emissions of the World's Richest People* (Oxfam GB for Oxfam International, November 2022).
93. Karl Marx and Friedrich Engels, *The Communist Manifesto* (Penguin Books, 2002), 223.
94. Robbie Davis-Floyd, Robin Lim, Vicki Penwell and Tsipy Ivry, 'Sustainable Birth Care in Disaster Zones and During Pandemics: Low-Tech, Skilled Touch', in *Sustainable Birth in Disruptive Times*, eds Kim Gutschow, Robbie Davis-Floyd and Betty-Anne Daviss (Springer, 2021), 261–276, 262.
95. Kim Gutschow, Robbie Davis-Floyd and Betty-Anne Daviss, 'Conclusion: Sustainable Maternity Care in Disruptive Times', in *Sustainable Birth in Disruptive Times*, eds Kim Gutschow, Robbie Davis-Floyd and Betty-Anne Daviss (Springer, 2021), 295–308, 296.
96. Vincanne Adams, Sienna R. Craig and Arlene Samen, 'Alternative Accounting in Maternal and Infant Global Health', *Global Public Health* 11, no. 3 (2016): 276–294, 288.

CHAPTER 7 FROM THE 'WOMB' OF THE PRESENT …

1. Karl Marx, 'Author's Preface' to *A Contribution to The Critique Of The Political Economy*, trans. N. I. Stone (e-artnow, 2019), paragraph 4.
2. Dervla Marphy, 'Foreword: The Family Experience of Home Birth', in *Untangling the Maternity Crisis*, eds Nadine Edwards, Rosemary Mander and Jo Murphy-Lawless (London and New York: Routledge, 2018), xiv–xx, xviii; original emphasis.

3. Fredric Jameson, *The Political Unconscious: Narrative as a Socially Symbolic Act* (London, Routledge: 1981), 102.
4. Silvia Federici, 'Introduction', in *Birth Work as Care Work: Stories from Activist Birth Communities*, ed. Alana Apfel (Oakland, CA: PM Press, 2016), xxi–xxv, xxii.
5. Jameson, *The Political Unconscious*, 102.
6. On 'no time to care' within the maternity service context see, for example, Fiona Dykes, '"No Time to Care": Midwifery Work on Postnatal Wards in England', in *Emotions in Midwifery and Reproduction*, eds Billie Hunter and Ruth Deery (Basingstoke, England: Palgrave Macmillan, 2009), 90–104.
7. On 'caring enough to strike', see Tithi Bhattacharya, 'Caring Enought to Strike: US Teachers' Strikes in Perspective' *RS21*, 22 January 2019, www.rs21.org.uk/2019/01/22/caring-enough-to-strike-us-teachers-strikes-in-perspective/ (last accessed May 2024).
8. Caitlin R. Williams, Celeste Jerez, Karen Klein, Malena Correa, José M. Belizán and Gabriela Cormick, 'Obstetric Violence: A Latin American Legal Response to Mistreatment During Childbirth', *British Journal of Obstetrics and Gynaecology* 125, no. 10 (2018): 1208–1211.
9. For further discussion of court cases, see for example, Betty-Anne Daviss, 'What Made Her Think She Could Win In Court? Models of Success in Seeking Justice Across Cultures in a Neoliberal World', in *Birthing Models on the Human Rights Frontier: Speaking Truth to Power*, eds Betty-Anne Daviss and Robbie Davis-Floyd (Routledge, 2020), 184-204; 'Human Rights in Maternity Care: The Key Facts', *Birthrights*, May 2021, https://birthrights.org.uk/factsheets/human-rights-in-maternity-care/#commonlaw (last accessed May 2024).
10. Chris Hendry, 'The New Zealand Maternity System: A Midwifery Renaissance', in *Birth Models That Work*, eds Robbie Davis-Floyd, Lesley Barclay, Betty-Anne Daviss and Jan Tritten (Berkeley: University of California Press, 2009), 55–87.
11. For a discussion of the model, see Celia P. Grigg and Sally K. Tracy, 'New Zealand's Unique Maternity System', *Women and Birth* 26, no. 1 (2013): e59–e64.
12. See, for example, Judith McAra-Couper, Andrea Gilkison, Susan Crowther, Marion Hunter, Claire Hotchin and Jackie Gunn, 'Partnership and Reciprocity with Women Sustain Lead Maternity Carer Midwives in Practice', *New Zealand College of Midwives Journal*, no. 49 (2014): 27–31.
13. Te Whatu Ora & Te Aka Whai Ora, *Health Workforce Plan 2023/24*, 4 July 2023 (Aotearoa New Zealand: Te Whatu Ora & Te Aka Whai Ora, 2023), www.tewhatuora.govt.nz/publications/health-workforce-plan-202324/ (last accessed May 2024).
14. See, for example, 'Te Ara ō Hine – Tapu Ora', Auckland University of Technology, 30 March 2021, https://www.aut.ac.nz/news/stories/te-ara-o-hine-tapu-ora (last accessed May 2024); Jean Te Huia, *Whaia Te Aronga a Ngā Kaiwhakawhānau Māori: The Māori Midwifery Workforce in Aotearoa* (Te Rau Ora, 2020).
15. Irihapeti Ramsden, *Kawa Whakaruruhau: Guidelines for Nursing and Midwifery Education* (Nursing Council of New Zealand, 19 February 1992).
16. Ibid., 7.

17. Julia Chinyere Oparah and Black Women Birthing Justice, 'Beyond Coercion and Malign Neglect: Black Women and the Struggle for Birth Justice', in *Birthing Justice: Black Women, Pregnancy, and Childbirth*, eds Julia Chinyere Oparah and Alicia D. Bonaparte (New York and London: Routledge, 2016), 1–18.
18. Ibid., 15.
19. Ibid.
20. Asteir Bey, Aimee Brill, Chanel Porchia-Albert, Melissa Gradilla and Nan Strauss, *Advancing Birth Justice: Community-Based Doula Models as a Standard of Care for Ending Racial Disparities* (United States: Ancient Song Doula Services; Village Birth International; Every Mother Counts, 25 March 2019), 8.
21. Ibid., 21.
22. Priscilla A. Ocen and Julia Chinyere Oparah, 'Beyond Shackling: Prisons, Pregnancy, and the Struggle for Birth Justice', in *Birthing Justice: Black Women, Pregnancy, and Childbirth*, eds Julia Chinyere Oparah and Alicia D. Bonaparte (New York and London: Routledge, 2016), 187–197, 196–197.
23. See, for example, Rebecca L. Bakal and Monica R. McLemore, 'Re/Envisioning Birth Work: Community-Based Doula Training for Low-Income and Previously Incarcerated Women in the United States', in *Sustainable Birth in Disruptive Times*, eds Kim Gutschow, Robbie Davis-Floyd and Betty-Anne Daviss (Springer, 2021), 85–98.
24. Ibid.
25. Bey et al., *Advancing Birth Justice*, 21.
26. Mama Glow Foundation, *Birth Worker Burnout: Exploring Integrative Approaches to Nurturing a Healthy Doula Workforce* (Mama Glow Foundation, n.d.), https://mamaglowfoundation.org/wp-content/uploads/2023/01/Birth_Worker_Burnout_Brief.pdf (last accessed May 2024).
27. Doula Sarah Davis, quoted in Bari Meltzer Norman and Barbara Katz Rothman, 'The New Arrival: Labor Doulas and the Fragmentation of Midwifery and Caregiving', in *Laboring On: Birth in Transition in the United States*, eds Wendy Simonds, Barbara Katz Rothman and Bari Meltzer Norman (Routledge, 2007), 251–282, 264.
28. Kira Neel, Roberta Goldman, Denise Marte, Gisel Bello and Melissa B. Nothnagle, 'Hospital-Based Maternity Care Practitioners' Perceptions of Doulas', *Birth* 46, no. 2 (2019): 355–361, 358.
29. See, for instance, Paula M. Kett, Marieke S. van Eijk, Grace A. Guenther and Susan M. Skillman, ''This Work that We're Doing is Bigger than Ourselves': A Qualitative Study with Community-based Birth Doulas in the United States', *Perspectives on Sexual and Reproductive Health* 54, no. 3 (2022): 99–108, 106.
30. Doula D., quoted in *Freebirth Stories*, eds Mavis Kirkham and Nadine Edwards(Sheffield: Birth Practice and Politics Forum, 2023), 258.
31. RCM Members Survey (England), conducted March 2023, reported on in 'RCM Survey of Midwives and MSWs in England: Overworked and Underpaid', Royal College of Midwives, www.rcm.org.uk/rcm-survey-of-midwives-and-msws-in-england/#:~:text=87%25%20of%20respondents%20across%20the,their%20workplace%20was%20safely%20staffed (last accessed May 2024).
32. Maddie McMahon, 'March with Midwives – Stand Together for Maternity Services', *Maternity & Midwifery Forum* (2022), https://maternityandmidwifery.

co.uk/march-with-midwives-stand-together-for-maternity-services/ (last accessed May 2024).

33. 'Midwives Haven', Association of Radical Midwives, www.midwifery.org.uk/midwives-haven/ (last accessed May 2024).
34. Ibid.
35. Laura Osman, 'Birth in Bomb Shelters: Ukrainian Midwives Look to Canada for Training', *CTV News*, 21 February 2023, www.ctvnews.ca/health/birth-in-bomb-shelters-ukrainian-midwives-look-to-canada-for-training-1.6281292 (last accessed May 2024).
36. Ibid.; See also 'Ukrainian-Canadian Midwife Supports Midwives in Ukraine; Emergency Skills and Association Recognition at the ICM Top of Agenda', *Association of Ontario Midwives*, https://tinyurl.com/2k8f6kkr (last accessed May 2024).
37. See, for example, 'Resistance is Fertile – Endorse Our Statement for Reproductive Justice for Palestine', *ReproSist*, 19 December 2023, https://tinyurl.com/yc4cvapr (last accessed May 2024).
38. 'Gaza: When Mothers Have to Bury At Least 7,700 Children, Very Basic Principles Are Being Challenged, UN Women's Rights Committee Says', United Nations/United Nations Human Rights Office of the High Commissioner, 16 February 2024, https://tinyurl.com/3u558wm9 (last accessed May 2024).
39. AJLabs, 'Israel-Gaza War in Maps and Charts: Live Tracker', *Aljazeera*, updated 30 May 2024, www.aljazeera.com/news/longform/2023/10/9/israel-hamas-war-in-maps-and-charts-live-tracker (last accessed May 2024); Adam Gaffney, 'Don't Believe the Conspiracies About the Gaza Death Toll', *The Nation*, 30 May 2024, www.thenation.com/article/world/gaza-death-toll-evidence/
40. ARC-Southeast, 'Letter: Reproductive Justice Includes Palestinian Liberation', ARC-Southeast, 24 October 2023, https://arc-southeast.org/2023/10/24/rj-includes-palestine/ (last accessed May 2024).
41. See, for example, Zena Chamas, 'Pregnant Mothers in Gaza Reportedly Facing Caesareans Without Anaesthetic, Emergency Hysterectomies and Death', *ABC*, 29 December 2023, www.abc.net.au/news/2023-12-29/being-pregnant-in-gaza-unsafe-women-paying-heaviest-price-in-war/103241724 (last accessed May 2024).
42. See, for example, Hiba Yazbek and Ameera Harouda, 'Thousands of Pregnant Women in Gaza Suffer from Malnutrition, Health Authorities Say', *The New York Times*, 10 March 2024, www.nytimes.com/2024/03/10/world/middleeast/gaza-malnutrition-hunger-pregnant-women.html (last accessed May 2024).
43. 'Resistance is Fertile – Endorse Our Statement for Reproductive Justice for Palestine', *ReproSist*.
44. See, for example, ICM, 'First Responders to the Climate Crisis: Caring for Fisherfolk on the Baba, Bhit, Shamspir and Salehabad Islands', *International Confederation of Midwives*, 12 December 2023, https://internationalmidwives.org/first-responders-to-the-climate-crisis-caring-for-fisherfolk-on-the-baba-bhit-shamspir-and-salehabad-islands/ (last accessed May 2024); Alison Reid, 'Fighting for Intergenerational Justice – Midwives Can Be Climate Champions', 17 January 2019, www.medact.org/2019/blogs/fighting-for-intergenerational-justice-midwives-can-be-climate-champions/ (last accessed May 2024).

45. David Harvey, 'History versus Theory: A Commentary on Marx's Method in Capital', *Historical Materialism* 20, no. 2 (2012): 3–38, 16.
46. Suellen Miller et al., 'Beyond Too Little, Too Late and Too Much, Too Soon: A Pathway Towards Evidence-Based, Respectful Maternity Care Worldwide', *The Lancet* 388, no. October 29 (2016): 2176–92.
47. Rebecca Ashley, Bahareh Goodarzi, Anna Horn, Hannah de Klerk, Susana E. Ku, Jason K Marcus, Kaveri Mayra, Fatimah Mohamied, Harriet Nayiga, Priya Sharma, Samson Udho, Madyasa Ruby Vijber and Rodante van der Waal, 'A Call for Critical Midwifery Studies: Confronting Systemic Injustice in Sexual, Reproductive, Maternal, and Newborn Care: Critical Midwifery Collective Writing Group', *Birth* 49, no. 3 (2022): 355–359, 358.
48. Rodante van der Waal, Kaveri Mayra, Anna Horn and Rachelle Chadwick, 'Obstetric Violence: An Intersectional Refraction through Abolition Feminism', *Feminist Anthropology* 4, no. 1 (2023): 91–114, 94.
49. As an example of an initiative involved in developing local worker cooperatives, see Cooperation Jackson, 'Who We Are', *Cooperation Jackson*, https://cooperationjackson.org/intro (last accessed May 2024).
50. See, for example, 'Poland: Women's Strike Against Abortion Law Amendment', *Amnesty International*, 3 October 2016, www.amnesty.nl/actueel/poland-womens-strike-against-abortion-law-amendment (last accessed May 2024); Egill Bjarnason, 'Women Across Iceland, Including the Prime Minister, Go On Strike For Equal Pay and No More Violence', *Associated Press*, 25 October 2023, https://apnews.com/article/iceland-women-strike-equal-pay-970669466116a2b1a5673a87337089d46 (last accessed May 2024); Claire Branigan and Cecelia Palmeiro, 'Women Strike in Latin America and Beyond', *NACLA*, 8 March 2018, https://nacla.org/news/2018/03/08/women-strike-latin-america-and-beyond (last accessed May 2024).
51. Cinzia Arruzza, Tithi Bhattacharya and Nancy Fraser, *Feminism for the 99%* (London: Verso, 2019), 5–10.
52. Ibid., 7; original emphasis.
53. Ibid., 8
54. 'A Women's Strike is impossible; that is why it is necessary', Verso Books blog, 7 March 2019, www.versobooks.com/en-gb/blogs/news/4246-a-women-s-strike-is-impossible-that-is-why-it-is-necessary (last accessed June 2024).
55. Simmonds notes that 'Kaiwhakawhānau is likely to be a relatively recent term or may be unique to some tribes. Tāpuhi … is also used to refer to traditional birth attendants.' Naomi Beth Simmonds, 'Tū Te Turuturu nō Hine-te-iwaiwa: Mana Wahine Geographies of Birth in Aotearoa New Zealand' (PhD Dissertation, University of Waikato, 2014), 225 [including footnote].
56. Christine M. Kenney, 'Midwives, Women and Their Families: A Māori Gaze: Towards Partnerships for Maternity Care in Aotearoa New Zealand', *AlterNative: An International Journal of Indigenous Peoples* 7, no. 2 (October 2011): 123–137, 126.
57. As outlined earlier, the word whānau is often translated into English as 'extended family', although the word has more expansive meaning than is indicated by that translation.
58. 'Midwife', in Julia Cresswell, *Oxford Dictionary of Word Origins* (Oxford University Press, 3rd edition, Online version, 2021).

59. The Care Collective, Andreas Chatzidakis, Jamie Hakim, Jo Littler, Catherine Rottenberg and Lynne Segal, *The Care Manifesto: The Politics of Interdependence* (London and New York: Verso, 2020), Chapter 2.
60. The Care Collective base the notion of promiscuous care on theory developed through AIDS activism, and in particular on work by Douglas Crimp. Ibid., Chapter 2; original emphasis.
61. Lynne Segal, 'Embedding Mothering at the Heart of Politics: Mamsie, Ten Years On', *Studies in the Maternal* 13, no. 1 (2020), 9.
62. Ibid.
63. 'Climate and Weather Related Disasters Surge Five-Fold Over 50 Years, But Early Warnings Save Lives – WMO report', *UN News*, 1 September 2020, https://news.un.org/en/story/2021/09/1098662 (last accessed May 2024).
64. Karl Marx, *Critique of the Gotha Programme* (Paris: Foreign Languages, 2021. Reprint of the first edition, Foreign Languages Press, Peking, 1972), 15.

GLOSSARY

1. World Health Organization, 'Maternal Deaths', *World Health Organization – The Global Health Observatory*, www.who.int/data/gho/indicator-metadata-registry/imr-details/4622 (last accessed May 2024).
2. World Health Organization, *Neonatal and Perinatal Mortality: Country, Regional and Global Estimates* (Geneva: World Health Organization, 2006): 6, https://iris.who.int/handle/10665/43444
3. World Health Organization, *Maternal and Perinatal Death Surveillance and Response: Materials to Support Implementation* (Geneva: World Health Organization, 2021): 6, https://iris.who.int/bitstream/handle/10665/348487/9789240036666-eng.pdf?sequence=1
4. Ibid., 6; original emphasis

Index

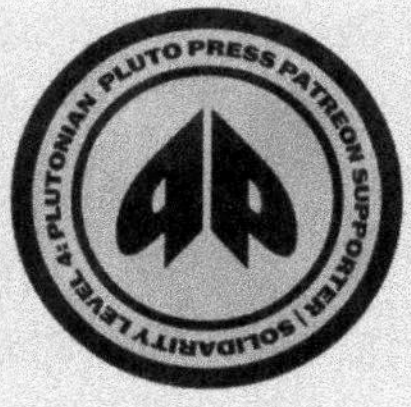

Thanks to our Patreon subscriber:

Ciaran Kane

Who has shown generosity and comradeship in support of our publishing.

Check out the other perks you get by subscribing to our Patreon – visit patreon.com/plutopress.

Subscriptions start from £3 a month.

The Pluto Press Newsletter

Hello friend of Pluto!

Want to stay on top of the best radical books we publish?

Then sign up to be the first to hear about our new books, as well as special events, podcasts and videos.

You'll also get 50% off your first order with us when you sign up.

Come and join us!

Go to bit.ly/PlutoNewsletter